SpringerBriefs in Statistics

SpringerBriefs present concise summaries of cutting-edge research and practical applications across a wide spectrum of fields. Featuring compact volumes of 50 to 125 pages, the series covers a range of content from professional to academic. Typical topics might include:

- A timely report of state-of-the art analytical techniques
- A bridge between new research results, as published in journal articles, and a contextual literature review
- A snapshot of a hot or emerging topic
- An in-depth case study or clinical example
- A presentation of core concepts that students must understand in order to make independent contributions

SpringerBriefs in Statistics showcase emerging theory, empirical research, and practical application in Statistics from a global author community.

SpringerBriefs are characterized by fast, global electronic dissemination, standard publishing contracts, standardized manuscript preparation and formatting guidelines, and expedited production schedules.

More information about this series at http://www.springer.com/series/8921

Stefan Bedbur • Udo Kamps

Multivariate Exponential Families: A Concise Guide to Statistical Inference

Springer

Stefan Bedbur
Institute of Statistics
RWTH Aachen University
Aachen, Germany

Udo Kamps
Institute of Statistics
RWTH Aachen University
Aachen, Germany

ISSN 2191-544X ISSN 2191-5458 (electronic)
SpringerBriefs in Statistics
ISBN 978-3-030-81899-9 ISBN 978-3-030-81900-2 (eBook)
https://doi.org/10.1007/978-3-030-81900-2

This Springer imprint is published by the registered company Springer Nature Switzerland AG.
The registered company address is: Gewerbestrasse 11, 6330 Cham, Switzerland

Preface

Parametric families of probability distributions and their properties are extensively studied in the literature on statistical modeling and inference. Exponential families of distributions comprise density functions of a particular form, which enables general assertions and leads to nice features. A literature review of books in the field of Mathematical Statistics discussing exponential families and their properties is given in the first chapter. With a focus on parameter estimation and hypotheses testing, we introduce the reader to properties of multivariate and multiparameter exponential families and show a variety of detailed examples. The material is widely self-contained and written in a mathematical setting. It may serve as a concise course on exponential families in a systematic structure. Supplements and comments can be found on the website https://www.isw.rwth-aachen.de/EF_SpringerBriefs.php.

Dear reader, we would very much appreciate receiving your remarks, criticism, and hints! We hope you will benefit from our introduction to exponential families.

Aachen, Germany
May 2021

Stefan Bedbur
Udo Kamps

Contents

1 **Introduction: Aims and Outline** 1

2 **Parametrizations and Basic Properties** 5
- 2.1 Definition and Examples 5
- 2.2 Order and Minimal Representation 17
- 2.3 Structural Properties and Natural Parametrization 23
- 2.4 Analytical Properties and Mean Value Parametrization 32

3 **Distributional and Statistical Properties** 43
- 3.1 Generating Functions 43
- 3.2 Marginal and Conditional Distributions 47
- 3.3 Product Measures 49
- 3.4 Sufficiency and Completeness 54
- 3.5 Score Statistic and Information Matrix 57
- 3.6 Divergence and Distance Measures 60

4 **Parameter Estimation** 65
- 4.1 Maximum Likelihood Estimation 66
- 4.2 Constrained Maximum Likelihood Estimation 71
- 4.3 Efficient Estimation 78
- 4.4 Asymptotic Properties 84

5 **Hypotheses Testing** 93
- 5.1 One-Sided Test Problems 93
- 5.2 Two-Sided Test Problems 101
- 5.3 Testing for a Selected Parameter 105
- 5.4 Testing for Several Parameters 109

6 **Exemplary Multivariate Applications** 117
- 6.1 Negative Multinomial Distribution 117
- 6.2 Dirichlet Distribution 125
- 6.3 Generalized Order Statistics 131

References 137

Index 141

Symbols

$\mathbb{N}$	$\{1, 2, 3, \ldots\}$ set of natural numbers
$\mathbb{N}_0$	$\{0, 1, 2, \ldots\}$ set of natural numbers including zero
$\mathbb{Z}$	$\{\ldots, -2, -1, 0, 1, 2, \ldots\}$ set of integers
$\mathbb{R}$	$(-\infty, \infty)$ set of real numbers
$\mathbb{C}$	$\{a + ib : a, b \in \mathbb{R}\}$ set of complex numbers
A^n	$\times_{i=1}^{n} A$ n-fold Cartesian product of set A
$\mathbb{1}_A$	indicator function of set A $\mathbb{1}_A(x) = 1$ if $x \in A$ and zero otherwise
$int(A)$	interior of set A
$\boldsymbol{a}^t$, $\mathbf{A}^t$	transpose of vector $\boldsymbol{a}$ and matrix $\mathbf{A}$
$\mathbf{A} > 0$ $(\mathbf{A} \geq 0)$	matrix $\mathbf{A}$ is positive (semi)definite
$\mathbf{A} \succeq \mathbf{B}$	matrix $\mathbf{A} - \mathbf{B}$ is positive semidefinite
∇g	$\left(\frac{\partial}{\partial x_1} g, \ldots, \frac{\partial}{\partial x_k} g\right)^t$ vector of partial derivatives (gradient) of $g : A \subset \mathbb{R}^k \to \mathbb{R}$
$\mathbf{H}_g$	$\left(\frac{\partial^2}{\partial x_i \partial x_j} g\right)_{1 \leq i,j \leq k}$ Hessian matrix of $g : A \subset \mathbb{R}^k \to \mathbb{R}$
$\mathbf{D}_g$	$(\nabla g_1, \ldots, \nabla g_n)^t$ Jacobian matrix of $g = (g_1, \ldots, g_n) : A \subset \mathbb{R}^k \to \mathbb{R}^n$
$(\mathcal{X}, \mathcal{B})$	measurable space of observations sample space $\mathcal{X}$ endowed with σ-algebra $\mathcal{B}$
$T : (\mathcal{X}, \mathcal{B}) \to (\mathcal{Y}, \mathcal{C})$	mapping $T : \mathcal{X} \to \mathcal{Y}$ is $(\mathcal{B} - \mathcal{C})$-measurable
$\mathbb{B}^k$	Borel sets of $\mathbb{R}^k$
$\mu_{\mathcal{X}}$	counting measure on the power set of $\mathcal{X}$
$\lambda_{\mathcal{X}}$	Lebesgue measure on the Borel sets of $\mathcal{X}$

$\mathfrak{poi}(\bullet)$	$\{\mathfrak{poi}(a) : a \in (0, \infty)\}$ family of Poisson distributions
$\mathfrak{b}(n_0, \bullet)$	$\{\mathfrak{b}(n_0, p) : p \in (0, 1)\}$ family of binomial distributions with $n_0 \in \mathbb{N}$ fixed
$\mathfrak{nb}(r_0, \bullet)$	$\{\mathfrak{nb}(r_0, p) : p \in (0, 1)\}$ family of negative binomial distributions with $r_0 \in \mathbb{N}$ fixed
$\mathfrak{geo}(\bullet)$	$\{\mathfrak{nb}(1, p) : p \in (0, 1)\}$ family of geometric distributions
$\mathfrak{kn}(\bullet, \bullet)$	$\{\mathfrak{kn}(\alpha, p) : \alpha \in (0, \infty), p \in (0, 1)\}$ family of Kemp discrete normal distributions
$\mathfrak{g}(\bullet, \bullet)$	$\{\mathfrak{g}(p, \tau) : p \in (0, 1), \tau \in \mathbb{R}\}$ family of Good distributions
$\mathfrak{m}(n_0, \bullet)$	$\{\mathfrak{m}(n_0, \boldsymbol{p}) : \boldsymbol{p} = (p_1, \ldots, p_k) \in (0, 1)^k, \sum_{i=1}^k p_i - 1\}$ family of multinomial distributions with $n_0 \in \mathbb{N}$ fixed
$\mathfrak{nm}(r_0, \bullet)$	$\{\mathfrak{nm}(r_0, \boldsymbol{p}) : \boldsymbol{p} = (p_1, \ldots, p_k) \in (0, 1)^k, \sum_{i=1}^k p_i < 1\}$ family of negative multinomial distributions with $r_0 \in \mathbb{N}$ fixed
$\mathfrak{mps}(h, \bullet)$	$\{\mathfrak{mps}(h, \boldsymbol{\vartheta}) : \boldsymbol{\vartheta} \in \Theta\}$ family of multivariate power series distributions with $\Theta \subset (0, \infty)^k$ and function h fixed
$\mathcal{N}(\bullet, \bullet)$	$\{\mathcal{N}(\mu, \sigma^2) : \mu \in \mathbb{R}, \sigma^2 \in (0, \infty)\}$ family of univariate normal distributions
$\mathcal{N}(\bullet, \sigma_0^2)$	$\{\mathcal{N}(\mu, \sigma_0^2) : \mu \in \mathbb{R}\}$ family of univariate normal distributions with $\sigma_0^2 \in (0, \infty)$ fixed
$\mathcal{N}(\mu_0, \bullet)$	$\{\mathcal{N}(\mu_0, \sigma^2) : \sigma^2 \in (0, \infty)\}$ family of univariate normal distributions with $\mu_0 \in \mathbb{R}$ fixed
$\mathcal{N}_k(\bullet, \boldsymbol{\Sigma}_0)$	$\{\mathcal{N}_k(\boldsymbol{\mu}, \boldsymbol{\Sigma}_0) : \boldsymbol{\mu} \in \mathbb{R}^k\}$ family of multivariate normal distributions with $\boldsymbol{\Sigma}_0 \in \mathbb{R}^{k \times k}$ fixed
$\mathcal{IN}(\bullet, \bullet)$	$\{\mathcal{IN}(\mu, \eta) : \mu, \eta \in (0, \infty)\}$ family of inverse normal distributions
$\mathcal{G}(\bullet, \bullet)$	$\{\mathcal{G}(\alpha, \beta) : \alpha, \beta \in (0, \infty)\}$ family of gamma distributions
$\mathcal{E}(\bullet)$	$\{\mathcal{G}(\alpha, 1) : \alpha \in (0, \infty)\}$ family of exponential distributions
$\mathcal{D}(\bullet)$	$\{\mathcal{D}(\boldsymbol{\beta}) : \boldsymbol{\beta} \in (0, \infty)^{k+1}\}$ family of Dirichlet distributions
$\mathcal{B}(\bullet, \bullet)$	$\{\mathcal{D}(\beta_1, \beta_2) : \beta_1, \beta_2 \in (0, \infty)\}$ family of beta distributions
$\mathcal{L}(h, \bullet)$	$\{\mathcal{L}(h, \boldsymbol{a}) : \boldsymbol{a} \in (0, \infty)^k\}$ family of Liouville distributions with function h fixed

Chapter 1
Introduction: Aims and Outline

The study of parametric families of probability distributions is a main foundation of statistical modeling and inference. Although some probability distributions may be quite different at first sight with respect to their density functions, they can be observed to share a similar structure and common nice properties. Such findings always motivate to look for explanations and to examine the reasons behind the similarities.

Let us take a look at three distributions to illustrate a starting point for the topic of exponential families.

A basic discrete, one-parameter distribution is the binomial distribution with counting density function

$$f_p(x) = \binom{n}{x} p^x (1-p)^{n-x}, \qquad x \in \{0, 1, \ldots, n\}, \tag{1.1}$$

for some fixed natural number n and parameter $p \in (0, 1)$.

An important continuous two-parameter distribution is the gamma distribution with Lebesgue density function

$$f_{\alpha,\beta}(x) = \frac{1}{\Gamma(\beta)\,\alpha^\beta} x^{\beta-1} \exp\left\{-\frac{x}{\alpha}\right\}, \qquad x \in (0, \infty), \tag{1.2}$$

and parameters $\alpha \in (0, \infty)$ and $\beta \in (0, \infty)$.

As a third distribution, we consider a multivariate normal distribution with Lebesgue density function

$$f_{\boldsymbol{\mu}}(\boldsymbol{x}) = \frac{1}{(2\pi)^{k/2}} \exp\left\{-\frac{1}{2}(\boldsymbol{x}-\boldsymbol{\mu})^t(\boldsymbol{x}-\boldsymbol{\mu})\right\}, \qquad \boldsymbol{x} \in \mathbb{R}^k, \tag{1.3}$$

S. Bedbur, U. Kamps, *Multivariate Exponential Families: A Concise Guide to Statistical Inference*, SpringerBriefs in Statistics,
https://doi.org/10.1007/978-3-030-81900-2_1

for $k \in \mathbb{N}$, its covariance matrix given by the k-dimensional unity matrix, and parameter vector $\boldsymbol{\mu} = (\mu_1, \ldots, \mu_k)^t \in \mathbb{R}^k$.

These distributions are different with respect to their support, dimension, and number of parameters.

On the other hand, by rewriting the density functions in formulas (1.1)–(1.3) according to

$$f_p(x) = (1-p)^n \exp\left\{\ln\left(\frac{p}{1-p}\right)x\right\}\binom{n}{x}, \tag{1.4}$$

$$f_{\alpha,\beta}(x) = \frac{1}{\Gamma(\beta)\,\alpha^\beta} \exp\left\{-\frac{x}{\alpha} + \beta\ln(x)\right\}\frac{1}{x}, \tag{1.5}$$

and

$$f_{\boldsymbol{\mu}}(\boldsymbol{x}) = \exp\left\{-\frac{\boldsymbol{\mu}^t\boldsymbol{\mu}}{2}\right\} \exp\left\{\sum_{j=1}^k \mu_j x_j\right\} \frac{\exp\{-\boldsymbol{x}^t\boldsymbol{x}/2\}}{(2\pi)^{k/2}}, \tag{1.6}$$

all of the density functions exhibit a common multiplicative structure

$$f_\vartheta(x) = C(\vartheta)\exp\left\{\sum_{j=1}^k Z_j(\vartheta)T_j(x)\right\} h(x), \qquad x \in \mathcal{X}, \tag{1.7}$$

where ϑ denotes the respective parameter (vector) and $\mathcal{X}$ is the support of the distribution. Here, the first factor $C(\vartheta)$ is a normalizing constant depending only on ϑ. In the exponent of the second factor, $Z_1(\vartheta), \ldots, Z_k(\vartheta)$ are constants depending only on ϑ, and $T_1, \ldots, T_k$ are mappings on $\mathcal{X}$, which are free of ϑ (with $k = 1$ in formula (1.4) and $k = 2$ in formula (1.5)). The third factor h is a function on $\mathcal{X}$ not depending on ϑ.

Distribution families with density functions of the form (1.7) are called *exponential families*. Having seen that the aforementioned distributions constitute exponential families (see formulas (1.4)–(1.6)), several questions arise at this point, such as the following:

- Are there other distributions (uni- and multivariate, one- and multiparameter distributions) possessing exponential family structure?
- What are special properties of an exponential family, and are there advantages when having statistical inference in mind?
- What is the use of a unified approach and a general theory of exponential families?

It will turn out that the exponential family structure comprises many well known distributions and that there are major benefits when considering exponential families of distributions in statistical inference. Various properties are found to hold true under fairly general assumptions on the underlying exponential family, which gives rise for a unified approach.

Exponential families are discussed in textbooks and monographs on Mathematical Statistics, usually. There are respective examples, recurring examples or chapters, such as in Bickel and Doksum [16], Ferguson [24], Keener [35], Kotz et al. [37, Chapter 54 by M. Casalis], Lehmann and Casella [39], Lehmann and Romano [40], Liese and Miescke [42], Lindsey [44], Pfanzagl [50], Shao [55] and Witting [63] or books dedicated to exponential families, such as the fundamental accounts of Brown [20], Jørgensen [29], Letac [41], Barndorff-Nielsen [4], and Sundberg [56]. In particular, the books of Witting [63] and Brown [20] influenced the present text on exponential families.

In the sequel, we focus on properties of multivariate and multiparameter exponential families along with a variety of detailed examples as well as on the use of exponential families in parameter estimation and hypotheses testing, mainly based on the maximum-likelihood principle. Nevertheless, the present introductory material also serves as a solid basis for other methods of statistical inference within exponential families.

Chapters 2–5 offer a widely self-contained, mathematically rigorous and concise course on exponential families in a systematic structure for Master- and Ph.D.-students. The text can be considered an introduction to Mathematical Statistics restricted to using exponential families. As prerequisites, the reader should have a solid knowledge of calculus, linear algebra, and of an introduction to probability and measure theory. For the chapter on hypotheses testing, a former introductory course on statistics may be helpful.

In Chaps. 2 and 3 on parametrizations, distributional and statistical properties of exponential families, the proofs of assertions are not detailed; however, ideas and references are given, throughout. Thereafter, in Chaps. 4 and 5 on parameter estimation and hypotheses testing within exponential families, proofs and derivations are worked out. In Chap. 6, three multiparameter and multivariate families of distributions are exemplarily examined in order to utilize and illustrate the results on exponential families, and, by this, the benefit of a general approach is demonstrated.

In the present concise introduction to multiparameter exponential families, several topics have been left out, such as the field of variance functions, cuts, advanced structural results, confidence regions, others than maximum-likelihood approaches, and Bayesian inference. For further reading on the theory and applications of exponential families, we refer to, for example, Brown [20], Lehmann and Casella [39], and Liese and Miescke [42] regarding Bayesian methods, Brown [20], Letac [41], Barndorff-Nielsen [4], Witting [63], Kotz et al. [37, Chapter 54] and Liese and Mieschke [42] regarding structural considerations and statistical inference, as well as to the recent monograph Sundberg [56] highlighting different fields of applications in statistics.

Chapter 2
Parametrizations and Basic Properties

2.1 Definition and Examples

Motivated by the examples in the introduction, we start with the formal definition of an exponential family by specifying the form of a probability density function.

Definition 2.1 Let $(\mathcal{X}, \mathcal{B})$ be a measurable space and $\mathcal{P} = \{P_\vartheta : \vartheta \in \Theta\}$ be a parametric family of probability distributions on $\mathcal{B}$, where $\Theta \neq \emptyset$ denotes a set of real parameters or parameter vectors. If there exist

- a σ-finite measure μ on $\mathcal{B}$ dominating $\mathcal{P}$,
- mappings $C, Z_1, \ldots, Z_k : \Theta \to \mathbb{R}$ and
- mappings $h, T_1, \ldots, T_k$: $(\mathcal{X}, \mathcal{B}) \to (\mathbb{R}^1, \mathbb{B}^1)$ with $h \geq 0$

for some integer $k \in \mathbb{N}$ in such a way that

$$f_\vartheta(x) = \frac{dP_\vartheta}{d\mu}(x) = C(\vartheta) \exp\left\{\sum_{j=1}^{k} Z_j(\vartheta)T_j(x)\right\} h(x), \qquad x \in \mathcal{X}, \tag{2.1}$$

is a μ-density of P_ϑ for every $\vartheta \in \Theta$, then $\mathcal{P}$ is said to form an *exponential family* (EF).

By the definition of the mappings involved in formula (2.1), the functions $C, Z_1, \ldots, Z_k$ do not depend on $x \in \mathcal{X}$, and the functions $h, T_1, \ldots, T_k$ do not depend on $\vartheta \in \Theta$.

S. Bedbur, U. Kamps, *Multivariate Exponential Families: A Concise Guide to Statistical Inference*, SpringerBriefs in Statistics,
https://doi.org/10.1007/978-3-030-81900-2_2

It is clear from the definition that an EF may have various different representations. The mappings $C, Z_1, \ldots, Z_k$ and $h, T_1, \ldots, T_k$ as well as the number k and the dominating measure μ in formula (2.1) are not uniquely determined. For instance, for some $j \in \{1, \ldots, k\}$, we may replace $Z_j(\vartheta)$ by $Z_j(\vartheta) - a$ and h by $h \exp\{aT_j\}$ for some constant $a \in \mathbb{R}$ to obtain another representation of the densities. Likewise, a shift of T_j and a respective modification of C gives a new representation. Moreover, although being artificial, setting $Z_{k+1} = 0$ or $T_{k+1} = 0$ yields another representation with $k+1$ summands in the exponent.

Since $\int f_\vartheta d\mu = 1$ for all $\vartheta \in \Theta$, $C(\vartheta)$ is just a normalizing constant.

Lemma 2.2 *In the situation of Definition 2.1, we have for every $\vartheta \in \Theta$*

$$0 < C(\vartheta) = \left[\int \exp\left\{ \sum_{j=1}^{k} Z_j(\vartheta) T_j(x) \right\} h(x)\, d\mu(x) \right]^{-1} < \infty .$$

Many well known univariate and multivariate distributions form EFs when varying one or more of their parameters. Here, the dominating measure μ is usually the counting measure (in the discrete case) or the Lebesgue measure (in the continuous case). We show some prominent examples; in particular, the distributions in the introduction turn out to form EFs when varying the parameters. Throughout the text, superscript t at a vector or matrix denotes transposition.

Examples: $\mathfrak{poi}(\bullet)$, $\mathfrak{b}(n_0, \bullet)$, $\mathfrak{nb}(r_0, \bullet)$, $\mathfrak{geo}(\bullet)$, $\mathfrak{En}(\bullet, \bullet)$, $\mathfrak{g}(\bullet, \bullet)$, $\mathfrak{m}(n_0, \bullet)$

In the following examples and throughout, let $\mu_{\mathcal{X}}$ denote the counting measure on the power set of $\mathcal{X}$.

Example 2.3 (Poisson Distribution) The counting density of the Poisson distribution $\mathfrak{poi}(a)$, $a \in (0, \infty)$, is given by

$$f_a(x) = e^{-a} \frac{a^x}{x!} = e^{-a} e^{\ln(a) x} \frac{1}{x!}, \qquad x \in \mathbb{N}_0 .$$

Hence, $\mathfrak{poi}(\bullet) = \{\mathfrak{poi}(a) : a \in (0, \infty)\}$ forms an EF with representation (2.1) given by $\mu = \mu_{\mathbb{N}_0}$, $k = 1$,

$$C(a) = e^{-a}, \qquad Z_1(a) = \ln(a), \qquad a \in (0, \infty),$$

$$\text{and} \qquad T_1(x) = x, \qquad h(x) = \frac{1}{x!}, \qquad x \in \mathbb{N}_0 .$$

Example 2.4 (Binomial Distribution) The counting density of the binomial distribution $\mathfrak{b}(n, p)$, $n \in \mathbb{N}$, $p \in (0, 1)$, is given by

$$f_{n,p}(x) = \binom{n}{x} p^x (1-p)^{n-x}$$

$$= (1-p)^n \exp\left\{\ln\left(\frac{p}{1-p}\right)x\right\} \binom{n}{x}, \qquad x \in \{0, 1, \ldots, n\} = \mathcal{X}.$$

Hence, for fixed $n = n_0 \in \mathbb{N}$, $\mathfrak{b}(n_0, \bullet) = \{\mathfrak{b}(n_0, p) : p \in (0, 1)\}$ forms an EF with representation (2.1) given by $\mu = \mu_{\mathcal{X}}$, $k = 1$,

$$C(p) = (1-p)^{n_0}, \qquad Z_1(p) = \ln\left(\frac{p}{1-p}\right), \qquad p \in (0, 1),$$

$$\text{and} \qquad T_1(x) = x, \qquad h(x) = \binom{n_0}{x}, \qquad x \in \mathcal{X}.$$

Example 2.5 (Negative Binomial Distribution) The counting density of the negative binomial distribution $\mathfrak{nb}(r, p)$, $r \in \mathbb{N}$, $p \in (0, 1)$, is given by

$$f_{r,p}(x) = \binom{x+r-1}{x} p^r (1-p)^x$$

$$= p^r e^{\ln(1-p)x} \binom{x+r-1}{x}, \qquad x \in \mathbb{N}_0.$$

Hence, for fixed $r = r_0 \in \mathbb{N}$, $\mathfrak{nb}(r_0, \bullet) = \{\mathfrak{nb}(r_0, p) : p \in (0, 1)\}$ forms an EF with representation (2.1) given by $\mu = \mu_{\mathbb{N}_0}$, $k = 1$,

$$C(p) = p^{r_0}, \qquad Z_1(p) = \ln(1-p), \qquad p \in (0, 1),$$

$$\text{and} \qquad T_1(x) = x, \qquad h(x) = \binom{x+r_0-1}{x}, \qquad x \in \mathbb{N}_0.$$

In particular, for $r_0 = 1$, the EF $\mathfrak{geo}(\bullet) = \mathfrak{nb}(1, \bullet)$ of *geometric distributions* results.

Example 2.6 (Kemp Discrete Normal Distribution) The counting density of the Kemp discrete normal distribution $\mathfrak{kn}(\alpha, p)$, $\alpha \in (0, \infty)$, $p \in (0, 1)$, is given by

$$f_{\alpha,p}(x) = \left(\sum_{j=-\infty}^{\infty} \alpha^j p^{j(j-1)/2} \right)^{-1} \alpha^x p^{x(x-1)/2}$$

$$= \left(\sum_{j=-\infty}^{\infty} \alpha^j p^{j(j-1)/2} \right)^{-1} \exp\left\{ \ln(\alpha)x + \ln(p)\frac{x(x-1)}{2} \right\}, \quad x \in \mathbb{Z}.$$

Hence, $\mathfrak{kn}(\bullet, \bullet) = \{\mathfrak{kn}(\alpha, p) : \alpha \in (0, \infty), p \in (0, 1)\}$ forms an EF with representation (2.1) given by $\mu = \mu_{\mathbb{Z}}$, $k = 2$,

$$C(\alpha, p) = \left(\sum_{j=-\infty}^{\infty} \alpha^j p^{j(j-1)/2} \right)^{-1}$$

$$Z_1(\alpha, p) = \ln(\alpha), \qquad Z_2(\alpha, p) = \ln(p), \qquad \alpha \in (0, \infty), \; p \in (0, 1),$$

and $$T_1(x) = x, \qquad T_2(x) = \frac{x(x-1)}{2}, \qquad h(x) = 1, \qquad x \in \mathbb{Z}.$$

Example 2.7 (Good Distribution) The counting density of the Good distribution $\mathfrak{g}(p, \tau)$, $p \in (0, 1)$, $\tau \in \mathbb{R}$, is given by

$$f_{p,\tau}(x) = \left(\sum_{j=1}^{\infty} p^j j^\tau \right)^{-1} p^x x^\tau$$

$$= \left(\sum_{j=1}^{\infty} p^j j^\tau \right)^{-1} \exp\{\ln(p)x + \tau \ln(x)\}, \qquad x \in \mathbb{N}.$$

Hence, $\mathfrak{g}(\bullet, \bullet) = \{\mathfrak{g}(p, \tau) : p \in (0, 1), \tau \in \mathbb{R}\}$ forms an EF with repre sentation (2.1) given by $\mu = \mu_{\mathbb{N}}$, $k = 2$,

$$C(p, \tau) = \left(\sum_{j=1}^{\infty} p^j j^\tau \right)^{-1}$$

$$Z_1(p, \tau) = \ln(p), \qquad Z_2(p, \tau) = \tau, \qquad p \in (0, 1), \; \tau \in \mathbb{R},$$

$$\text{and} \quad T_1(x) = x\,, \quad T_2(x) = \ln(x)\,, \quad h(x) = 1\,, \quad x \in \mathbb{N}\,.$$

Example 2.8 (Multinomial Distribution) The counting density of the multinomial distribution $\mathfrak{m}(n, \boldsymbol{p})$, $n \in \mathbb{N}$, $\boldsymbol{p} = (p_1, \ldots, p_k)^t \in \Theta = \{(q_1, \ldots, q_k)^t \in (0, 1)^k : \sum_{i=1}^k q_i = 1\}$, where $k \geq 2$, is given by

$$\begin{aligned} f_{n,\boldsymbol{p}}(\boldsymbol{x}) &= \frac{n!}{\prod_{i=1}^k x_i!} \left(\prod_{j=1}^k p_j^{x_j} \right) \\ &= \exp\left\{ \sum_{j=1}^k \ln(p_j) x_j \right\} \frac{n!}{\prod_{i=1}^k x_i!} \end{aligned}$$

for $\boldsymbol{x} = (x_1, \ldots, x_k)^t \in \mathcal{X} = \{(y_1, \ldots, y_k)^t \in \mathbb{N}_0^k : \sum_{i=1}^k y_i = n\}$. Hence, for fixed $n = n_0 \in \mathbb{N}$, $\mathfrak{m}(n_0, \bullet) = \{\mathfrak{m}(n_0, \boldsymbol{p}) : \boldsymbol{p} \in \Theta\}$ forms an EF with representation (2.1) given by $\mu = \mu_{\mathcal{X}}$,

$$C(\boldsymbol{p}) = 1\,, \quad Z_j(\boldsymbol{p}) = \ln(p_j)\,, \quad \boldsymbol{p} \in \Theta\,,$$

$$\text{and} \quad T_j(\boldsymbol{x}) = x_j\,, \quad h(\boldsymbol{x}) = \frac{n_0!}{\prod_{i=1}^k x_i!}\,, \quad \boldsymbol{x} \in \mathcal{X}\,, \quad 1 \leq j \leq k\,.$$

More examples of discrete multivariate EFs can be found in [28, pp. 12–16] including, among others, the family of multivariate power series distributions. The negative multinomial distribution, which forms a particular multivariate power series distribution, is studied in Sect. 6.1.

Remark 2.9 A general class of discrete multivariate distributions is given by *multivariate power series distributions* with counting densities of the form

$$f_{\boldsymbol{\vartheta}}(\boldsymbol{x}) = C(\boldsymbol{\vartheta})\, h(\boldsymbol{x}) \prod_{j=1}^k \vartheta_j^{x_j}\,, \qquad \boldsymbol{x} = (x_1, \ldots, x_k)^t \in \mathcal{X} \subset \mathbb{N}_0^k\,, \tag{2.2}$$

where h is an appropriate function, $\boldsymbol{\vartheta} = (\vartheta_1, \ldots, \vartheta_k)^t \in \Theta \subset (0, \infty)^k$ is a parameter vector, and $C(\boldsymbol{\vartheta})$ is a normalizing constant (see [28, Chapter 38]). We denote the multivariate power series distribution with density function (2.2) by $\mathfrak{mps}(h, \boldsymbol{\vartheta})$. For fixed function h, $\mathfrak{mps}(h, \bullet) = \{\mathfrak{mps}(h, \boldsymbol{\vartheta}) : \boldsymbol{\vartheta} \in \Theta\}$ forms an EF.

Examples of particular distributions contained in the class of multivariate power series distributions are the multinomial distribution (see Example 2.8), the negative multinomial distribution (see Sect. 6.1), the multivariate logarithmic series distribution ($C(\boldsymbol{\vartheta}) = -1/\ln(1-\sum_{j=1}^{k}\vartheta_j)$, $\boldsymbol{\vartheta} \in (0,1)^k$ with $\sum_{j=1}^{k}\vartheta_j < 1$, and $h(\boldsymbol{x}) = (\sum_{j=1}^{k} x_j - 1)!/\prod_{j=1}^{k} x_j!$, $\boldsymbol{x} \in \mathbb{N}_0^k \setminus \{(0,\ldots,0)^t\}$), and the joint distribution of k independent Poisson-distributed random variables (see Example 2.3).

Examples: $\mathcal{N}(\bullet,\bullet)$, $\mathcal{N}(\mu_0,\bullet)$, $\mathcal{N}(\bullet,\sigma_0^2)$, $\mathcal{IN}(\bullet,\bullet)$, $\mathcal{G}(\bullet,\bullet)$, $\mathcal{E}(\bullet)$, $\mathcal{D}(\bullet)$, $\mathcal{B}(\bullet,\bullet)$

In the following examples and throughout, let $\lambda_{\mathcal{X}}$ denote the Lebesgue measure on the Borel sets of $\mathcal{X}$.

Example 2.10 (Normal Distribution) The Lebesgue density of the normal distribution $\mathcal{N}(\mu,\sigma^2)$ with mean $\mu \in \mathbb{R}$ and variance $\sigma^2 \in (0,\infty)$ is given by

$$f_{\mu,\sigma^2}(x) = \frac{1}{\sqrt{2\pi\sigma^2}} \exp\left\{-\frac{(x-\mu)^2}{2\sigma^2}\right\}$$

$$= \frac{1}{\sqrt{\sigma^2}} \exp\left\{-\frac{\mu^2}{2\sigma^2}\right\} \exp\left\{\frac{\mu x}{\sigma^2} - \frac{x^2}{2\sigma^2}\right\} \frac{1}{\sqrt{2\pi}}, \qquad x \in \mathbb{R}.$$

Hence, $\mathcal{N}(\bullet,\bullet) = \{\mathcal{N}(\mu,\sigma^2) : \mu \in \mathbb{R}, \sigma^2 \in (0,\infty)\}$ forms an EF with representation (2.1) given by $\mu = \lambda_{\mathbb{R}}$, $k = 2$,

$$C(\mu,\sigma^2) = \frac{1}{\sqrt{\sigma^2}} \exp\left\{-\frac{\mu^2}{2\sigma^2}\right\},$$

$$Z_1(\mu,\sigma^2) = \frac{\mu}{\sigma^2}, \qquad Z_2(\mu,\sigma^2) = -\frac{1}{2\sigma^2}, \qquad \mu \in \mathbb{R},\ \sigma^2 \in (0,\infty),$$

and $\quad T_1(x) = x, \qquad T_2(x) = x^2, \qquad h(x) = \frac{1}{\sqrt{2\pi}}, \qquad x \in \mathbb{R}.$

Moreover, when fixing either $\mu = \mu_0$ or $\sigma^2 = \sigma_0^2$, the classes $\mathcal{N}(\mu_0,\bullet) = \{\mathcal{N}(\mu_0,\sigma^2) : \sigma^2 \in (0,\infty)\}$ and $\mathcal{N}(\bullet,\sigma_0^2) = \{\mathcal{N}(\mu,\sigma_0^2) : \mu \in \mathbb{R}\}$ are easily seen to form one-parameter EFs.

By choosing $\alpha = \exp\{-(1-2\mu)/(2\sigma^2)\}$ and $p = \exp\{-1/\sigma^2\}$ in Example 2.6 (cf. [26, p. 475]), the Kemp distribution $\mathfrak{kn}(\alpha, p)$ is seen to be a discrete version of the normal distribution $\mathcal{N}(\mu,\sigma^2)$.

Example 2.11 (Inverse Normal Distribution) The Lebesgue density of the inverse normal distribution $\mathcal{IN}(\mu, \eta)$, $\mu, \eta \in (0, \infty)$, is given by

$$\begin{aligned} f_{\mu,\eta}(x) &= \sqrt{\frac{\eta}{2\pi x^3}} \exp\left\{-\frac{\eta(x-\mu)^2}{2\mu^2 x}\right\} \\ &= \sqrt{\eta} \exp\left\{\frac{\eta}{\mu}\right\} \exp\left\{-\frac{\eta x}{2\mu^2} - \frac{\eta}{2x}\right\} \sqrt{\frac{1}{2\pi x^3}}, \qquad x \in (0, \infty). \end{aligned}$$

Hence, $\mathcal{IN}(\bullet, \bullet) = \{\mathcal{IN}(\mu, \eta) : \mu, \eta \in (0, \infty)\}$ forms an EF with representation (2.1) given by $\mu = \lambda_{(0,\infty)}$, $k = 2$,

$$C(\mu, \eta) = \sqrt{\eta} \exp\left\{\frac{\eta}{\mu}\right\},$$

$$Z_1(\mu, \eta) = -\frac{\eta}{2\mu^2}, \qquad Z_2(\mu, \eta) = -\frac{\eta}{2}, \qquad \mu, \eta \in (0, \infty),$$

and $$T_1(x) = x, \qquad T_2(x) = \frac{1}{x}, \qquad h(x) = \sqrt{\frac{1}{2\pi x^3}}, \qquad x \in (0, \infty).$$

Example 2.12 (Gamma Distribution) The Lebesgue density of the gamma distribution $\mathcal{G}(\alpha, \beta)$, $\alpha, \beta \in (0, \infty)$, is given by

$$\begin{aligned} f_{\alpha,\beta}(x) &= \frac{1}{\Gamma(\beta)\,\alpha^\beta}\, x^{\beta-1} \exp\left\{-\frac{x}{\alpha}\right\} \\ &= \frac{1}{\Gamma(\beta)\,\alpha^\beta} \exp\left\{-\frac{x}{\alpha} + \beta \ln(x)\right\} \frac{1}{x}, \qquad x \in (0, \infty). \end{aligned}$$

Hence, $\mathcal{G}(\bullet, \bullet) = \{\mathcal{G}(\alpha, \beta) : \alpha, \beta \in (0, \infty)\}$ forms an EF with representation (2.1) given by $\mu = \lambda_{(0,\infty)}$, $k = 2$,

$$C(\alpha, \beta) = \frac{1}{\Gamma(\beta)\,\alpha^\beta}, \quad Z_1(\alpha, \beta) = -\frac{1}{\alpha}, \quad Z_2(\alpha, \beta) = \beta, \quad \alpha, \beta \in (0, \infty),$$

and $$T_1(x) = x, \qquad T_2(x) = \ln(x), \qquad h(x) = \frac{1}{x}, \qquad x \in (0, \infty).$$

Fixing $\beta = 1$, the resulting *exponential distributions* $\mathcal{E}(\alpha)$, $\alpha \in (0, \infty)$, form the one-parameter EF $\mathcal{E}(\bullet) = \{\mathcal{G}(\alpha, 1) : \alpha \in (0, \infty)\}$ with representation (2.1) given by $\mu = \lambda_{(0,\infty)}$, $k = 1$,

$$C(\alpha) = \frac{1}{\alpha}, \qquad Z_1(\alpha) = -\frac{1}{\alpha}, \qquad \alpha \in (0, \infty),$$

$$\text{and} \qquad T_1(x) = x\,, \qquad h(x) = 1\,, \qquad x \in (0, \infty)\,.$$

By choosing $\alpha = 2$ and $\beta = n/2$, we arrive at the EF $\{\chi^2(n) : n \in \mathbb{N}\} = \{\mathcal{G}(2, n/2) : n \in \mathbb{N}\}$ of *chi-square distributions*.

For $p = \exp\{-1/\alpha\}$ and $\tau = \beta - 1$, the Good distribution $\mathfrak{g}(p, \tau)$ in Example 2.7 (cf. [26, p. 530]) is seen to be a discrete version of the gamma distribution $\mathcal{G}(\alpha, \beta)$.

Example 2.13 (Dirichlet Distribution) The Lebesgue density of the Dirichlet distribution $\mathcal{D}(\boldsymbol{\beta})$, $\boldsymbol{\beta} = (\beta_1, \ldots, \beta_{k+1})^t \in (0, \infty)^{k+1}$, is given by

$$f_{\boldsymbol{\beta}}(\boldsymbol{x}) = \frac{1}{B(\boldsymbol{\beta})} \left(\prod_{j=1}^{k} x_j^{\beta_j - 1} \right) \left(1 - \sum_{j=1}^{k} x_j \right)^{\beta_{k+1} - 1}$$

$$= \frac{1}{B(\boldsymbol{\beta})} \exp\left\{ \left(\sum_{j=1}^{k} \beta_j \ln(x_j) \right) + \beta_{k+1} \ln\left(1 - \sum_{j=1}^{k} x_j \right) \right\} \left[\left(1 - \sum_{j=1}^{k} x_j \right) \prod_{j=1}^{k} x_j \right]^{-1}$$

for $\boldsymbol{x} = (x_1, \ldots, x_k)^t \in \mathcal{X} = \{(y_1, \ldots, y_k)^t \in (0, 1)^k : \sum_{i=1}^{k} y_i < 1\}$, where $B(\boldsymbol{\beta}) = [\prod_{i=1}^{k+1} \Gamma(\beta_i)]/\Gamma(\sum_{i=1}^{k+1} \beta_i)$ denotes the beta function evaluated at $\boldsymbol{\beta}$. Hence, $\mathcal{D}(\bullet) = \{\mathcal{D}(\boldsymbol{\beta}) : \boldsymbol{\beta} \in (0, \infty)^{k+1}\}$ and, in particular, by setting $k = 1$, the family $\mathcal{B}(\bullet, \bullet) = \{\mathcal{D}(\beta_1, \beta_2) : \beta_1, \beta_2 \in (0, \infty)\}$ of *beta distributions* are seen to form EFs. The EF of Dirichlet distributions is studied in Sect. 6.2.

Further continuous univariate EFs are given by the family of *log-normal distributions* and the family of *inverse gamma distributions*. Other examples of continuous multivariate distributions, which lead to multiparameter EFs, are multivariate normal distributions, particular multivariate Liouville distributions, and *Wishart distributions* (for the latter, see, e.g., [37, pp. 662/663] and [36, Section 2.4]).

Remark 2.14 A general class of continuous multivariate distributions is given by so-called *Liouville distributions* with Lebesgue density functions proportional to

$$h\left(\sum_{j=1}^{k} x_j \right) \prod_{j=1}^{k} x_j^{a_j - 1}\,, \qquad x_1, \ldots, x_k > 0\,, \tag{2.3}$$

where h is an appropriate non-negative function and $a_1, \ldots, a_k$ are positive parameters (see [37, Chapter 50] and [47, Section 8.5] for details). We denote the Liouville distribution with density function (2.3) by $\mathcal{L}(h, (a_1, \ldots, a_k)^t)$. Obviously, for fixed h, $\mathcal{L}(h, \bullet) = \{\mathcal{L}(h, \boldsymbol{a}) : \boldsymbol{a} \in (0, \infty)^k\}$ then forms an EF. An EF structure may also arise if h depends on additional parameters as the following two examples show.

For $h(y) = y^{\beta-1}\exp\{-y/\alpha\}$, $y > 0$, with positive parameters α and β, the resulting Liouville distribution (of the first kind) has density function

$$\frac{\Gamma(a_\bullet)}{\Gamma(a_\bullet + \beta - 1)\,(\prod_{j=1}^{k}\Gamma(a_j))\,\alpha^{a_\bullet+\beta-1}}\left(\sum_{j=1}^{k} x_j\right)^{\beta-1}\prod_{j=1}^{k} x_j^{a_j-1}\,e^{-x_j/\alpha}$$

for $x_1, \ldots, x_k > 0$, where $a_\bullet = \sum_{i=1}^{k} a_i$. The particular case $\beta = 1$ yields the joint density function of k independent gamma-distributed random variables with common scale parameter α (see Example 2.12).

Choosing $h(y) = (1-y)^{\beta-1}$ for $0 < y < 1$ (zero otherwise) and some $\beta > 0$, we obtain the Dirichlet distribution $\mathcal{D}(a_1, \ldots, a_k, \beta)$ defined on the open simplex $\{(x_1, \ldots, x_k)^t \in (0,1)^k : \sum_{i=1}^{k} x_i < 1\}$ (see Example 2.13) as a particular Liouville distribution (of the second kind).

The function h in Definition 2.1 is free of ϑ and, indeed, as we will later see, it does not play a role in statistical inference. As a $(\mathcal{B} - \mathbb{B}^1)$-measurable non-negative mapping, h may be considered a μ-density of a measure ν, i.e., we have $\nu(A) = \int h\mathbb{1}_A\,d\mu$, $A \in \mathcal{B}$, where $\mathbb{1}_A$ denotes the indicator function of the set A. For short, we write $\nu = h\mu$ in that case. Since μ is σ-finite and h is real-valued, ν is then σ-finite as well (see, e.g., [6, pp. 104/105]). We may therefore absorb h into the dominating measure to obtain a shorter representation of the EF.

Lemma 2.15 *Let $\mathcal{P}$ be an EF with representation (2.1), and let $\nu = h\mu$ be the measure with μ-density h. Then, for every $\vartheta \in \Theta$, a ν-density of P_ϑ is given by*

$$g_\vartheta(x) = \frac{dP_\vartheta}{d\nu}(x) = C(\vartheta)\exp\left\{\sum_{j=1}^{k} Z_j(\vartheta)T_j(x)\right\}, \qquad x \in \mathcal{X}. \tag{2.4}$$

Remark 2.16 In formula (2.4), we have $g_\vartheta > 0$ for every $\vartheta \in \Theta$, which implies that ν and P_ϑ are equivalent measures, i.e., $\nu(N) = 0$ if and only if $P_\vartheta(N) = 0$ is valid for every $N \in \mathcal{B}$. As a consequence, all distributions in an EF are necessarily equivalent. In particular, the *support* of P_ϑ, defined by

$$supp(P_\vartheta) = \{x \in \mathcal{X} : f_\vartheta(x) > 0\}$$

for the discrete case and by

$$supp(P_\vartheta) = \{x \in \mathcal{X} : P_\vartheta(V) > 0 \text{ for all open sets } V \subset \mathcal{X} \text{ with } x \in V\}$$

for the continuous case, does not depend on ϑ. By fixing some parameter $\vartheta_0 \in \Theta$, this allows for a further representation of the EF given by the P_{ϑ_0}-densities

$$\frac{dP_\vartheta}{dP_{\vartheta_0}}(x) = \frac{C(\vartheta)}{C(\vartheta_0)} \exp\left\{\sum_{j=1}^{k}(Z_j(\vartheta) - Z_j(\vartheta_0))\, T_j(x)\right\}, \qquad x \in \mathcal{X},$$

for $\vartheta \in \Theta$.

By Remark 2.16, a necessary condition for a family of distributions to form an EF is that all distributions have the same support. Counterexamples are therefore near at hand. For instance, the continuous uniform distribution on the interval $[a, b]$, $-\infty < a < b < \infty$, does not form an EF when a or b are supposed to vary. Another counterexample is provided by the two-parameter exponential distribution with varying location parameter. Both distribution families are examples for so-called *truncated EFs*, which have also been studied in the literature. For a recent work on estimation in truncated EFs, we refer to [1].

For the sake of a short notation, we introduce the (column) vectors $\boldsymbol{Z} = (Z_1, \ldots, Z_k)^t$ and $\boldsymbol{T} = (T_1, \ldots, T_k)^t$ of parameter functions and statistics, respectively. Then, for $\vartheta \in \Theta$ and $x \in \mathcal{X}$, $\boldsymbol{Z}(\vartheta)^t \boldsymbol{T}(x) = \sum_{j=1}^{k} Z_j(\vartheta) T_j(x)$ is the scalar product of $\boldsymbol{Z}(\vartheta)$ and $\boldsymbol{T}(x)$.

Moreover, let $P_\vartheta^{\boldsymbol{T}}$ denote the distribution of $\boldsymbol{T}$ under P_ϑ being defined on the Borel sets $\mathbb{B}^k$ of $\mathbb{R}^k$, i.e., $P_\vartheta^{\boldsymbol{T}}(A) = P_\vartheta(\boldsymbol{T}^{-1}(A))$, $A \in \mathbb{B}^k$. By an integral transformation, it is easily seen that if $\mathcal{P} = \{P_\vartheta : \vartheta \in \Theta\}$ forms an EF so do the image distributions $P_\vartheta^{\boldsymbol{T}}$, $\vartheta \in \Theta$, of $\boldsymbol{T}$ (see, e.g., [39, pp. 31/32] or [63, p. 149]).

Lemma 2.17 *Let $\mathcal{P}$ be an EF with representation (2.4), and let $\nu^{\boldsymbol{T}}(A) = \nu(\boldsymbol{T}^{-1}(A))$, $A \in \mathbb{B}^k$, denote the image measure of ν under $\boldsymbol{T}$. Then, for every $\vartheta \in \Theta$, a $\nu^{\boldsymbol{T}}$-density of $P_\vartheta^{\boldsymbol{T}}$ is given by*

$$g_\vartheta^{\boldsymbol{T}}(\boldsymbol{t}) = \frac{dP_\vartheta^{\boldsymbol{T}}}{d\nu^{\boldsymbol{T}}}(\boldsymbol{t}) = C(\vartheta) \exp\left\{\boldsymbol{Z}(\vartheta)^t \boldsymbol{t}\right\}, \qquad \boldsymbol{t} = (t_1, \ldots, t_k)^t \in \mathbb{R}^k,$$

and $\mathcal{P}^{\boldsymbol{T}} = \{P_\vartheta^{\boldsymbol{T}} : \vartheta \in \Theta\}$ forms an EF.

Note that the measure $\nu^{\boldsymbol{T}}$ in Lemma 2.17 is σ-finite, since $0 < g_\vartheta^{\boldsymbol{T}} < \infty$ and $\int g_\vartheta^{\boldsymbol{T}} d\nu^{\boldsymbol{T}} = 1 < \infty$ for $\vartheta \in \Theta$ (see, e.g., [6, pp. 98/99]).

Example: $\mathcal{N}_k(\bullet, \boldsymbol{\Sigma}_0)$

Example 2.18 (Multivariate Normal Distribution) The Lebesgue density of the multivariate normal distribution $\mathcal{N}_k(\boldsymbol{\mu}, \boldsymbol{\Sigma})$ with mean vector $\boldsymbol{\mu} \in \mathbb{R}^k$ and positive definite covariance matrix $\boldsymbol{\Sigma} \in \mathbb{R}^{k\times k}$ is given by

$$f_{\boldsymbol{\mu},\boldsymbol{\Sigma}}(\boldsymbol{x}) = \frac{1}{(2\pi)^{k/2}\sqrt{\det(\boldsymbol{\Sigma})}} \exp\left\{-\frac{1}{2}\,||\boldsymbol{x}-\boldsymbol{\mu}||_{\boldsymbol{\Sigma}}^2\right\}, \qquad \boldsymbol{x} \in \mathbb{R}^k,$$

$$\text{where} \qquad ||\boldsymbol{y}||_{\boldsymbol{\Sigma}} = \sqrt{\boldsymbol{y}^t\,\boldsymbol{\Sigma}^{-1}\,\boldsymbol{y}}, \qquad \boldsymbol{y} \in \mathbb{R}^k,$$

denotes the Mahalanobis norm with weight matrix $\boldsymbol{\Sigma}^{-1}$. For fixed $\boldsymbol{\Sigma} = \boldsymbol{\Sigma}_0$, $\mathcal{P} = \mathcal{N}_k(\bullet, \boldsymbol{\Sigma}_0) = \{\mathcal{N}_k(\boldsymbol{\mu}, \boldsymbol{\Sigma}_0) : \boldsymbol{\mu} \in \mathbb{R}^k\}$ forms an EF with representation (2.1) given by $\mu = \lambda_{\mathbb{R}^k} = \lambda^k$, say,

$$C(\boldsymbol{\mu}) = \exp\left\{-\frac{||\boldsymbol{\mu}||_{\boldsymbol{\Sigma}_0}^2}{2}\right\}, \qquad \boldsymbol{Z}(\boldsymbol{\mu}) = \boldsymbol{\mu}, \qquad \boldsymbol{\mu} \in \mathbb{R}^k,$$

$$\text{and} \qquad \boldsymbol{T}(\boldsymbol{x}) = \boldsymbol{\Sigma}_0^{-1}\boldsymbol{x}, \qquad h(\boldsymbol{x}) = \frac{\exp\left\{-||\boldsymbol{x}||_{\boldsymbol{\Sigma}_0}^2/2\right\}}{(2\pi)^{k/2}\sqrt{\det(\boldsymbol{\Sigma}_0)}}, \qquad \boldsymbol{x} \in \mathbb{R}^k.$$

Now, let $\nu = h\lambda^k = \mathcal{N}_k(\boldsymbol{0}, \boldsymbol{\Sigma}_0)$. For $A \in \mathbb{B}^k$, an integral transformation then yields

$$\begin{aligned}
\nu^{\boldsymbol{T}}(A) &= \nu(\boldsymbol{T}^{-1}(A)) = \int_{\boldsymbol{T}^{-1}(A)} h(\boldsymbol{x})\,d\lambda^k(\boldsymbol{x})\\
&= \int_A h(\boldsymbol{\Sigma}_0\boldsymbol{u})\,|\det(\boldsymbol{\Sigma}_0)|\,d\lambda^k(\boldsymbol{u}) = \int_A f_{\boldsymbol{0},\boldsymbol{\Sigma}_0^{-1}}(\boldsymbol{u})\,d\lambda^k(\boldsymbol{u}).
\end{aligned}$$

Hence, $\nu^{\boldsymbol{T}} = \mathcal{N}_k(\boldsymbol{0}, \boldsymbol{\Sigma}_0^{-1})$. By Lemma 2.17, the distribution of $\boldsymbol{T}$ under $P_{\boldsymbol{\mu}}$ is given by

$$\begin{aligned}
P_{\boldsymbol{\mu}}^{\boldsymbol{T}}(A) &= \int_A C(\boldsymbol{\mu})\,e^{\boldsymbol{Z}(\boldsymbol{\mu})^t\boldsymbol{t}}\,d\nu^{\boldsymbol{T}}(\boldsymbol{t})\\
&= \int_A C(\boldsymbol{\mu})\,e^{\boldsymbol{\mu}^t\boldsymbol{t}}\,f_{\boldsymbol{0},\boldsymbol{\Sigma}_0^{-1}}(\boldsymbol{t})\,d\lambda^k(\boldsymbol{t}) = \int_A f_{\boldsymbol{\Sigma}_0^{-1}\boldsymbol{\mu},\boldsymbol{\Sigma}_0^{-1}}(\boldsymbol{t})\,d\lambda^k(\boldsymbol{t}),
\end{aligned}$$

i.e., $P_{\boldsymbol{\mu}}^{\boldsymbol{T}} = \mathcal{N}_k(\boldsymbol{\Sigma}_0^{-1}\boldsymbol{\mu}, \boldsymbol{\Sigma}_0^{-1})$, for $\boldsymbol{\mu} \in \mathbb{R}^k$. Hence, $\mathcal{P}^{\boldsymbol{T}} = \mathcal{N}_k(\bullet, \boldsymbol{\Sigma}_0^{-1})$, here.

In general, however, the dominating measure $\nu^{\boldsymbol{T}}$ of $\mathcal{P}^{\boldsymbol{T}}$ in Lemma 2.17 will have a complicated structure. For instance, in case of the EF $\mathcal{N}(\bullet, \bullet)$ in Example 2.10, we have $\boldsymbol{T}(x) = (x, x^2)^t$, $x \in \mathbb{R}$, and, since $\nu^{\boldsymbol{T}}$ and $P_{\vartheta}^{\boldsymbol{T}}$ are equivalent by Remark 2.16, $supp(\nu^{\boldsymbol{T}}) = \{(x, x^2)^t : x \in \mathbb{R}\}$, i.e., the support of $\nu^{\boldsymbol{T}}$ is given by the graph of the standard parabola in the plane. In particular, $supp(\nu^T)$ has no inner points, and ν^T does not have a Lebesgue density.

Remark 2.19 As the preceding examples show, the concept of the EF is rich and allows for a unifying study of various different distributions. It comprises univariate, one-parameter distributions, such as $\mathfrak{poi}(\bullet)$ and $\mathcal{E}(\bullet)$ shown in Examples 2.3 and 2.12, as well as multivariate, multiparameter distributions as, for instance, $\mathfrak{m}(n_0, \bullet)$ and $\mathcal{D}(\bullet)$ in Examples 2.8 and 2.13. Examples for univariate EFs with more than one parameter are provided by $\mathfrak{kn}(\bullet, \bullet)$ and $\mathcal{N}(\bullet, \bullet)$ in Examples 2.6 and 2.10. Finally, multivariate, one-parameter EFs appear in a natural way when sampling from a univariate, one-parameter EF (see Sect. 3.3); a particular example is the family $\{\mathcal{N}_k((\mu, \ldots, \mu)^t, \mathbf{E}_k) : \mu \in \mathbb{R}\}$, where $\mathbf{E}_k$ denotes the k-dimensional unit matrix.

Many of the aforementioned examples of EFs will be considered again and studied in more detail in the sequel. An overview is provided in Table 2.1.

Table 2.1 EFs discussed in this book listed by type and number of parameters

Type	Parameters	EF	Discussed in ...
Discrete	1	$\mathfrak{poi}(\bullet)$	Examples 2.3, 2.37, 2.64, 3.2, 3.14, 3.22, 3.31, 4.7, 4.28, 5.6
	1	$\mathfrak{b}(n_0, \bullet)$	Examples 2.4, 2.38, 2.57, 3.3, 3.22, 4.8, 4.28
	1	$\mathfrak{nb}(r_0, \bullet)$	Examples 2.5, 2.51, 3.22, 3.32, 4.28
	1	$\mathfrak{geo}(\bullet)$	Examples 2.5, 2.51, 3.22, 3.32, 4.28
	2	$\mathfrak{kn}(\bullet, \bullet)$	Example 2.6
	2	$\mathfrak{g}(\bullet, \bullet)$	Examples 2.7, 3.23
	k (≥2)	$\mathfrak{m}(n_0, \bullet)$	Examples 2.8, 2.46, 3.4, 3.24
	k (≥2)	$\mathfrak{nm}(r_0, \bullet)$	Section 6.1
	k (≥2)	$\mathfrak{mps}(h, \bullet)$	Remark 2.9
Continuous	1	$\mathcal{E}(\bullet)$	Examples 2.12, 3.10, 3.22, 4.28, 5.9
	1	$\mathcal{N}(\bullet, \sigma_0^2)$	Examples 2.10, 3.16, 5.7
	1	$\mathcal{N}(\mu_0, \bullet)$	Example 2.10
	2	$\mathcal{N}(\bullet, \bullet)$	Examples 2.10, 2.27, 2.31, 2.39, 2.52, 2.59, 3.5, 3.15, 3.25, 3.33, 4.9, 4.15
	2	$\mathcal{IN}(\bullet, \bullet)$	Examples 2.11, 2.25, 2.41, 2.58
	2	$\mathcal{G}(\bullet, \bullet)$	Examples 2.12, 2.24, 2.40, 2.53, 3.6, 3.23, 3.34, 4.24
	2	$\mathcal{B}(\bullet, \bullet)$	Example 2.13, Section 6.2
	k (≥ 2)	$\mathcal{N}_k(\bullet, \mathbf{\Sigma}_0)$	Examples 2.18, 2.28, 2.54, 2.65, 3.7, 3.16, 3.26, 3.35, 3.41, 4.10, 4.25, 5.14, 5.18
	k (≥ 2)	$\mathcal{D}(\bullet)$	Example 2.13, Section 6.2
	k (≥ 2)	$\mathcal{L}(h, \bullet)$	Remark 2.14

2.2 Order and Minimal Representation

For both, mathematical and practical reasons, a representation (2.1) of the EF in Definition 2.1 is desired, where the number k of summands is minimum. On the one hand, this will ensure that the parameter $\vartheta \in \Theta$ is identifiable meaning that different parameters correspond to different distributions in the EF. On the other hand, the vector $\boldsymbol{T}$ of statistics, which plays an important role in statistical inference, should have a dimension as small as possible. First, we define what is meant by a minimal representation of the EF.

Definition 2.20 Let $\mathcal{P}$ be an EF with representation (2.1). Then, $\mathcal{P}$ is said to have *order* k if the following implication holds true:

If $\tilde{\mu}$ is a σ-finite measure on $\mathcal{B}$, $\tilde{k} \in \mathbb{N}$, and if there are mappings $\tilde{C}, \tilde{Z}_1, \ldots, \tilde{Z}_{\tilde{k}} : \Theta \to \mathbb{R}$, and $\tilde{h}, \tilde{T}_1, \ldots, \tilde{T}_{\tilde{k}} : (\mathcal{X}, \mathcal{B}) \to (\mathbb{R}^1, \mathbb{B}^1)$ with $\tilde{h} \geq 0$ such that

$$\tilde{f}_\vartheta(x) = \frac{dP_\vartheta}{d\tilde{\mu}}(x) = \tilde{C}(\vartheta) \exp\left\{\sum_{j=1}^{\tilde{k}} \tilde{Z}_j(\vartheta)\tilde{T}_j(x)\right\} \tilde{h}(x), \qquad x \in \mathcal{X}, \tag{2.5}$$

is a $\tilde{\mu}$-density of P_ϑ for every $\vartheta \in \Theta$, then $\tilde{k} \geq k$.

In that case, we write $ord(\mathcal{P}) = k$, and representation (2.1) is said to be *minimal*.

Definition 2.20 is not suitable to determine the order of an EF in a given situation. Aiming for necessary and sufficient conditions for an EF to have order k, we introduce affine independence of mappings.

Definition 2.21 Let $\mathcal{Y} \neq \emptyset$ be a set, $k \in \mathbb{N}$, and $u_1, \ldots, u_k : \mathcal{Y} \to \mathbb{R}$ be mappings.

(a) $u_1, \ldots, u_k$ are called *affinely independent* if, for any $a_0, a_1, \ldots, a_k \in \mathbb{R}$,

$$a_0 + \sum_{j=1}^{k} a_j\, u_j(y) = 0 \quad \text{for all } y \in \mathcal{Y}$$

implies that $a_0 = a_1 = \cdots = a_k = 0$.

(continued)

Definition 2.21 (continued)
(b) Let $(\mathcal{Y}, \mathcal{C})$ be a measurable space, Q be a measure on $\mathcal{C}$, and $u_1, \ldots, u_k$ be $(\mathcal{C} - \mathbb{B}^1)$-measurable. Then, $u_1, \ldots, u_k$ are called *Q-affinely independent* if $\tilde{u}_1, \ldots, \tilde{u}_k : N^c \to \mathbb{R}$ are affinely independent in the sense of (a) for every $N \in \mathcal{C}$ with $Q(N) = 0$.

The following lemma connects the concepts of affine independence of mappings and linear independence of vectors in $\mathbb{R}^k$. A proof can be found in the web appendix.

Lemma 2.22 *Let $\mathcal{Y} \neq \emptyset$ be a set, $k \in \mathbb{N}$, and $u_1, \ldots, u_k : \mathcal{Y} \to \mathbb{R}$ be mappings. Moreover, let $\boldsymbol{u} = (u_1, \ldots, u_k) : \mathcal{Y} \to \mathbb{R}^k$ and $y_0 \in \mathcal{Y}$. Then, the following assertions are equivalent:*

(a) $u_1, \ldots, u_k$ are affinely independent.
(b) There exist $y_1, \ldots, y_k \in \mathcal{Y}$ such that $\boldsymbol{u}(y_1) - \boldsymbol{u}(y_0), \ldots, \boldsymbol{u}(y_k) - \boldsymbol{u}(y_0)$ are linearly independent (in $\mathbb{R}^k$).

Given representation (2.4) of an EF, it is clear that if $Z_1, \ldots, Z_k$ are not affinely independent or if $T_1, \ldots, T_k$ are not ν-affinely independent, the exponent in the densities can be reduced by a summand under respective modifications of C or ν. Hence, affine independence of $Z_1, \ldots, Z_k$ and ν-affine independence of $T_1, \ldots, T_k$ is a necessary condition for the EF to have order k. Indeed, the condition is also sufficient (see, e.g., [4, p. 113]). A detailed proof can be found, for instance, in [63, pp. 145/146].

Theorem 2.23 *Let $\mathcal{P}$ be an EF with representation (2.4). Then, the following assertions are equivalent:*

(a) $ord(\mathcal{P}) = k$,
(b) $Z_1, \ldots, Z_k$ are affinely independent and $T_1, \ldots, T_k$ are ν-affinely independent.

Note that, by Remark 2.16, ν-affine independence coincides with P_ϑ-affine independence for every $\vartheta \in \Theta$.

Examples: $\mathcal{G}(\bullet, \bullet)$, $\mathcal{IN}(\bullet, \bullet)$

Example 2.24 Consider the representation of $\mathcal{G}(\bullet, \bullet)$ in Example 2.12 with $Z_1(\alpha, \beta) = -1/\alpha$, $Z_2(\alpha, \beta) = \beta$ for $\alpha, \beta \in (0, \infty)$, and $T_1(x) = x$, $T_2(x) = \ln(x)$ for $x \in (0, \infty)$. Let

$$a_0 - \frac{a_1}{\alpha} + a_2\beta = 0 \qquad \text{for all } \alpha, \beta \in (0, \infty).$$

For $\alpha \to \infty$ and $\beta \to 0$, this gives $a_0 = 0$. Then, choosing $(\alpha, \beta) = (1, 1)$ and $(\alpha, \beta) = (1, 2)$ yields that $a_2 = 0$ and, thus, $a_1 = 0$. Hence, Z_1 and Z_2 are affinely independent. Now, suppose that T_1 and T_2 are not ν-affinely independent. Then, there exists a vector $(a_0, a_1, a_2) \neq (0, 0, 0)$ with

$$a_0 + a_1 x + a_2 \ln(x) = 0 \qquad \nu\text{-almost everywhere } (\nu\text{-a.e.}) .$$

For $x \to \infty$, the left-hand side tends to either $-\infty$ or ∞ and is therefore not equal to 0 on the interval (M, ∞) for some $M > 0$. Since $\nu((M, \infty)) > 0$, this forms a contradiction. Hence, T_1 and T_2 are ν-affinely independent, and we have $ord(\mathcal{G}(\bullet, \bullet)) = 2$ by Theorem 2.23. In particular, the representation is minimal.

Example 2.25 Consider the representation of $\mathcal{IN}(\bullet, \bullet)$ in Example 2.11 with

$$Z_1(\boldsymbol{\vartheta}) = -\frac{\eta}{2\mu^2}, \quad Z_2(\boldsymbol{\vartheta}) = -\frac{\eta}{2}, \quad \boldsymbol{\vartheta} = (\mu, \eta)^t \in (0, \infty)^2 ,$$

and $T_1(x) = x$, $T_2(x) = 1/x$ for $x \in (0, \infty)$. Setting $\boldsymbol{\vartheta}_0 = (\sqrt{2}, 4)^t$, $\boldsymbol{\vartheta}_1 = (1, 2)^t$, and $\boldsymbol{\vartheta}_2 = (1, 4)^t$, we obtain that

$$\mathbf{Z}(\boldsymbol{\vartheta}_1) - \mathbf{Z}(\boldsymbol{\vartheta}_0) = (-1, -1)^t - (-1, -2)^t = (0, 1)^t$$

$$\text{and} \qquad \mathbf{Z}(\boldsymbol{\vartheta}_2) - \mathbf{Z}(\boldsymbol{\vartheta}_0) = (-2, -2)^t - (-1, -2)^t = (-1, 0)^t$$

are linearly independent in $\mathbb{R}^2$. Hence, Z_1 and Z_2 are affinely independent by Lemma 2.22. Now, suppose that T_1 and T_2 are not ν-affinely independent. Then, there exists a vector $(a_0, a_1, a_2) \neq (0, 0, 0)$ with

$$a_0 + a_1 x + \frac{a_2}{x} = 0 \qquad \nu\text{-a.e.},$$

or, equivalently,

$$a_1 x^2 + a_0 x + a_2 = 0 \qquad \nu\text{-a.e.}.$$

This quadratic equation has at most two positive solutions x_1 and x_2, say. Since $\nu(\{x_1, x_2\}) = 0$, we have a contradiction. Hence, T_1 and T_2 are ν-affinely independent, and we obtain $ord(\mathcal{IN}(\bullet, \bullet)) = 2$ from Theorem 2.23. In particular, the representation is minimal.

To check for a representation of $\mathcal{P}$ to be minimal, the following equivalence is often useful. The assertion is obvious from the general rule $\boldsymbol{a}^t \mathbf{Cov}(\boldsymbol{U})\boldsymbol{a} = Var(\boldsymbol{a}^t \boldsymbol{U})$ for a random vector $\boldsymbol{U}$ and a constant vector $\boldsymbol{a}$, which implies that $\boldsymbol{a}^t \mathbf{Cov}(\boldsymbol{U})\boldsymbol{a} = 0$ if and only if $\boldsymbol{a}^t \boldsymbol{U}$ is almost surely (a.s.) constant (see also [63, pp. 145/146]).

Lemma 2.26 *Let $(\mathcal{Y}, \mathcal{C})$ be a measurable space, Q be a probability measure on $\mathcal{C}$, and $\boldsymbol{U} = (U_1, \ldots, U_k)^t : (\mathcal{Y}, \mathcal{C}) \rightarrow (\mathbb{R}^k, \mathbb{B}^k)$ a random vector with $E(U_j^2) < \infty$, $1 \leq j \leq k$. Then, the following assertions are equivalent:*

(a) $U_1, \ldots, U_k$ are Q-affinely independent.
(b) $\mathbf{Cov}(\boldsymbol{U}) > 0$, i.e., the covariance matrix of $\boldsymbol{U}$ is positive definite.

Examples: $\mathcal{N}(\bullet, \bullet)$, $\mathcal{N}_k(\bullet, \boldsymbol{\Sigma}_0)$

Example 2.27 Consider the representation of $\mathcal{N}(\bullet, \bullet)$ in Example 2.10 with

$$Z_1(\boldsymbol{\vartheta}) = \frac{\mu}{\sigma^2}, \quad Z_2(\boldsymbol{\vartheta}) = -\frac{1}{2\sigma^2}, \quad \boldsymbol{\vartheta} = (\mu, \sigma^2)^t \in \mathbb{R} \times (0, \infty),$$

and $T_1(x) = x$, $T_2(x) = x^2$, for $x \in \mathbb{R}$. Setting $\boldsymbol{\vartheta}_0 = (0, 1)^t$, $\boldsymbol{\vartheta}_1 = (0, 1/2)^t$, and $\boldsymbol{\vartheta}_2 = (1/2, 1/2)^t$, we obtain that

$$\begin{aligned} \boldsymbol{Z}(\boldsymbol{\vartheta}_1) - \boldsymbol{Z}(\boldsymbol{\vartheta}_0) &= (0, -1/2)^t \\ \text{and} \qquad \boldsymbol{Z}(\boldsymbol{\vartheta}_2) - \boldsymbol{Z}(\boldsymbol{\vartheta}_0) &= (1, -1/2)^t \end{aligned}$$

are linearly independent in $\mathbb{R}^2$. Hence, Z_1 and Z_2 are affinely independent by Lemma 2.22. Moreover, the covariance matrix of $\boldsymbol{T}(X) = (X, X^2)^t$ for $X \sim Q = \mathcal{N}(0, 1)$ is given by

$$\mathbf{Cov}_Q(\boldsymbol{T}) = \begin{pmatrix} 1 & 0 \\ 0 & 2 \end{pmatrix} > 0.$$

Thus, T_1 and T_2 are ν-affinely independent by Lemma 2.26 and Remark 2.16. Applying Theorem 2.23 then yields that $ord(\mathcal{N}(\bullet, \bullet)) = 2$. In particular, the representation is minimal.

Example 2.28 Consider the representation of $\mathcal{N}_k(\bullet, \boldsymbol{\Sigma}_0)$ in Example 2.18 with $\boldsymbol{Z}(\boldsymbol{\mu}) = \boldsymbol{\mu}$, $\boldsymbol{\mu} \in \mathbb{R}^k$, and $\boldsymbol{T}(\boldsymbol{x}) = \boldsymbol{\Sigma}_0^{-1}\boldsymbol{x}$, $\boldsymbol{x} \in \mathbb{R}^k$. If $a_0 \in \mathbb{R}$ and $\boldsymbol{a} \in \mathbb{R}^k$ are such that $a_0 + \boldsymbol{a}^t\boldsymbol{\mu} = 0$ for all $\boldsymbol{\mu} \in \mathbb{R}^k$, it directly follows that $a_0 = 0$ and $\boldsymbol{a} = \boldsymbol{0}$. Hence, $Z_1, \ldots, Z_k$ are affinely independent. Moreover, for every $\boldsymbol{\mu} \in \mathbb{R}^k$, $\mathbf{Cov}_{\boldsymbol{\mu}}(\boldsymbol{T}) = \boldsymbol{\Sigma}_0^{-1} > 0$ such that $T_1, \ldots, T_k$ are ν-affinely independent by Lemma 2.26. Applying Theorem 2.23 then yields that $ord(\mathcal{N}_k(\bullet, \boldsymbol{\Sigma}_0)) = k$. In particular, the representation is minimal.

In a minimal representation of an EF, the vectors $\boldsymbol{Z}$ and $\boldsymbol{T}$ of parameter functions and statistics, respectively, are uniquely determined up to non-degenerated affine transformations (see [4, p. 112]); a detailed proof is provided in [63, pp. 145–147].

Theorem 2.29 *Let $\mathcal{P}$ be an EF with minimal representations (2.1) and (2.5), i.e., $k = ord(\mathcal{P}) = \tilde{k}$. Then, there exist regular matrices $\mathbf{L}, \mathbf{M} \in \mathbb{R}^{k\times k}$ and vectors $\boldsymbol{l}, \boldsymbol{m} \in \mathbb{R}^k$ with*

$$\boldsymbol{Z} = \mathbf{L}\tilde{\boldsymbol{Z}} + \boldsymbol{l} \quad \text{and} \quad \boldsymbol{T} = \mathbf{M}\tilde{\boldsymbol{T}} + \boldsymbol{m} \quad \nu\text{-a.e.},$$

where $\tilde{\boldsymbol{Z}} = (\tilde{Z}_1, \ldots, \tilde{Z}_k)^t$ and $\tilde{\boldsymbol{T}} = (\tilde{T}_1, \ldots, \tilde{T}_k)^t$.

Finding a minimal representation for a given EF is an important step when aiming at statistical inference. Among others, it may ensure that the parameter $\vartheta \in \Theta$ is identifiable. Alternatively, in the literature, the identifiability property is ascribed to the set Θ of parameters or to the parametric family $\mathcal{P}$ of distributions.

Lemma 2.30 *Let $\mathcal{P}$ be an EF with representation (2.4). If $\boldsymbol{Z}$ is one-to-one and $T_1, \ldots, T_k$ are ν-affinely independent, then the parameter $\vartheta \in \Theta$ is identifiable, i.e., the mapping $\vartheta \mapsto P_\vartheta$, $\vartheta \in \Theta$, is one-to-one.*

Proof Let $P_{\vartheta_1} = P_{\vartheta_2}$ for $\vartheta_1, \vartheta_2 \in \Theta$. Then, we have $g_{\vartheta_1} = g_{\vartheta_2}$ ν-a.e., which is equivalent to

$$(\boldsymbol{Z}(\vartheta_1) - \boldsymbol{Z}(\vartheta_2))^t \boldsymbol{T} = \ln\left(\frac{C(\vartheta_2)}{C(\vartheta_1)}\right) \qquad \nu\text{-a.e.}.$$

Hence, we have $\boldsymbol{Z}(\vartheta_1) = \boldsymbol{Z}(\vartheta_2)$ by using that $T_1, \ldots, T_k$ are ν-affinely independent. Since $\boldsymbol{Z}$ is one-to-one, it follows that $\vartheta_1 = \vartheta_2$. □

In many applications, the parameters of some EF are supposed to satisfy certain constraints. This assumption leads to subfamilies which, of course, form EFs. The order of these embedded EFs may be smaller than or equal to the order of the original EF. We give a classical example (see [35, pp. 85–87]).

Example: Subfamilies of $\mathcal{N}(\bullet, \bullet)$

Example 2.31 Let $\mathcal{P} = \mathcal{N}(\bullet, \bullet)$ with representation as in Example 2.10, and recall that $ord(\mathcal{P}) = 2$ (see Example 2.27).

(a) First, we consider the subfamily $\mathcal{P}_1 = \{\mathcal{N}(\mu, \mu) : \mu \in (0, \infty)\}$ of $\mathcal{P}$. Setting $\sigma^2 = \mu$ in the density of $\mathcal{N}(\mu, \sigma^2)$, it is easily seen that $\mathcal{P}_1$ forms an EF with representation (2.1) given by $k = 1$,

$$C(\mu) = \frac{1}{\sqrt{\mu}} \exp\left\{-\frac{\mu}{2}\right\}, \qquad Z_1(\mu) = -\frac{1}{2\mu}, \qquad \mu \in (0, \infty),$$

and $T_1(x) = x^2, \quad h(x) = \frac{1}{\sqrt{2\pi}} e^x, \quad x \in \mathbb{R}.$

Hence, $\mathrm{ord}(\mathcal{P}_1) = 1$.

(b) Now, let $\mathcal{P}_2 = \{\mathcal{N}(\mu, \mu^2) : \mu \in \mathbb{R} \setminus \{0\}\}$. Replacing σ^2 by μ^2 in the density of $\mathcal{N}(\mu, \sigma^2)$, we arrive at a representation (2.1) of $\mathcal{P}_2$ given by $k = 2$,

$$C(\mu) = \frac{1}{\sqrt{\mu^2}}, \quad Z_1(\mu) = \frac{1}{\mu}, \quad \text{and} \quad Z_2(\mu) = -\frac{1}{2\mu^2}, \quad \mu \in \mathbb{R} \setminus \{0\},$$

and $h(x) = \frac{1}{\sqrt{2\pi e}}, \quad T_1(x) = x, \quad \text{and} \quad T_2(x) = x^2, \quad x \in \mathbb{R}.$

Since $\mathbf{Z}(1) - \mathbf{Z}(-1) = (2, 0)^t$ and $\mathbf{Z}(1/2) - \mathbf{Z}(-1) = (3, -3/2)^t$, Z_1 and Z_2 are affinely independent by Lemma 2.22. As shown in Example 2.27, T_1 and T_2 are $\mathcal{N}(0, 1)$-affinely independent and thus also $\mathcal{N}(1, 1)$-affinely independent. Hence, we have $ord(\mathcal{P}_2) = 2$ by Theorem 2.23.

Although both EFs, $\mathcal{P}_1$ and $\mathcal{P}_2$, in Example 2.31 are one-parameter subfamilies of $\mathcal{N}(\bullet, \bullet)$, their orders are different. When imposing the constraint for the parameters, the mappings Z_1 and Z_2 in Example 2.27 are no longer affinely independent in case (a) but they are in case (b). $\mathcal{P}_2$ forms an example for a so-called curved EF. We give a fairly general definition of the concept to keep it short, here (see [50, p. 28]); other definitions in the literature impose additional regularity conditions as, e.g., continuous second derivatives of $\mathbf{Z}$ on Θ, where Θ is assumed to be an open subset of $\mathbb{R}^m$ with $m < k$.

Definition 2.32 Let $\mathcal{P}$ be an EF with representation (2.1). If $Z_1, \ldots, Z_k$ are affinely independent and $int(\mathbf{Z}(\Theta)) = \emptyset$, i.e., the interior of $\mathbf{Z}(\Theta)$ is empty, then $\mathcal{P}$ is called a *curved* EF.

The statistical literature on curved EFs is vast; among others, geometrical aspects, inference, and applications, e.g., in graphical models and networks, have widely been studied. In the sequel, several properties of curved EFs are addressed while the main focus is on EFs with parameter spaces containing at least some inner points. More results on curved EFs can be found, for instance, in [20, 2, 5, 39, 44, 35, 56].

2.3 Structural Properties and Natural Parametrization

In Lemma 2.2, we have pointed out that the term $C(\vartheta)$ in representation (2.1) is just a normalizing constant. Moreover, it depends on ϑ only via $\mathbf{Z}(\vartheta) \in \mathbf{Z}(\Theta) = \{\mathbf{Z}(\vartheta) : \vartheta \in \Theta\}$. This finding allows for a more natural parametrization of the EF.

Definition 2.33 Let $\mathcal{P}$ be an EF with representation (2.1). The *natural parameter space* is defined by

$$\Xi^* = \{\boldsymbol{\zeta} = (\zeta_1, \ldots, \zeta_k)^t \in \mathbb{R}^k : 0 < \int \exp\left\{\sum_{j=1}^{k} \zeta_j T_j(x)\right\} h(x)\, d\mu(x) < \infty\}.$$

Note that the natural parameter space depends on representation (2.1) of the EF. Evidently, we have that $\mathbf{Z}(\Theta) \subset \Xi^*$. Moreover, by using the Hölder inequality, Ξ^* is readily seen to be convex; for a detailed proof, see [40, p. 48].

Theorem 2.34 *Let $\mathcal{P}$ be an EF with representation (2.1). Then, Ξ^* is a convex set in $\mathbb{R}^k$, i.e., if $\boldsymbol{\zeta}, \boldsymbol{\eta} \in \Xi^*$ and $\alpha \in [0, 1]$, then $\alpha\boldsymbol{\zeta} + (1 - \alpha)\boldsymbol{\eta} \in \Xi^*$.*

The natural parametrization of the EF and related notions are now introduced as follows.

Definition 2.35 Let $\mathcal{P}$ be an EF with representation (2.1), and let $\Xi = \mathbf{Z}(\Theta)$. The *natural parametrization* $P^*_{\boldsymbol{\zeta}}$, $\boldsymbol{\zeta} \in \Xi$, of $\mathcal{P}$ is defined by the μ-densities

$$f^*_{\boldsymbol{\zeta}}(x) = \frac{dP^*_{\boldsymbol{\zeta}}}{d\mu}(x) = C^*(\boldsymbol{\zeta}) \exp\left\{\sum_{j=1}^{k} \zeta_j T_j(x)\right\} h(x), \qquad x \in \mathcal{X}, \tag{2.6}$$

with normalizing constant $C^*(\boldsymbol{\zeta})$ for $\boldsymbol{\zeta} \in \Xi$. Formula (2.6) is also referred to as *canonical representation* of $\mathcal{P}$. Moreover, $\mathcal{P}$ is called

- full if $\Xi = \Xi^*$, and
- regular if $\Xi = \Xi^*$ and Ξ^* is open.

Remark 2.36 Following Lemma 2.15, a ν-density of P^*_{ζ} in Definition 2.35 is given by

$$g^*_{\zeta}(x) = \frac{dP^*_{\zeta}}{d\nu}(x) = C^*(\zeta) \exp\left\{\sum_{j=1}^{k} \zeta_j T_j(x)\right\}, \qquad x \in \mathcal{X},$$

for $\boldsymbol{\zeta} \in \Xi$; moreover, by Lemma 2.17, a $\nu^{\boldsymbol{T}}$-density of the image distribution $(P^*_{\zeta})^{\boldsymbol{T}}$ of $\boldsymbol{T} = (T_1, \ldots, T_k)^t$ is represented by

$$(g^*_{\zeta})^{\boldsymbol{T}}(\boldsymbol{t}) = \frac{d(P^*_{\zeta})^{\boldsymbol{T}}}{d\nu^{\boldsymbol{T}}}(\boldsymbol{t}) = C^*(\boldsymbol{\zeta})\, e^{\boldsymbol{\zeta}^t \boldsymbol{t}}, \qquad \boldsymbol{t} \in \mathbb{R}^k, \tag{2.7}$$

for $\boldsymbol{\zeta} \in \Xi$. A full EF with densities (2.7), which moreover satisfies that $int(\Xi^*) \neq \emptyset$ and that $\nu^{\boldsymbol{T}}$ is not concentrated on an affine hyperplane of $\mathbb{R}^k$, is referred to as *natural* EF (with *generating measure* $\nu^{\boldsymbol{T}}$) in the literature (see, e.g., [37, Chapter 54], and the references therein).

The natural parametrization of the EF is more convenient for inferential purposes and leads to various useful statistical properties. If exponential distributions are introduced by the Lebesgue density functions $\lambda \exp\{-\lambda x\}, x > 0$, for parameter $\lambda > 0$, then the respective EF is already given in natural parametrization with $\lambda \in \Xi = (0, \infty)$. The natural parametrization for the class $\mathcal{N}_k(\bullet, \boldsymbol{\Sigma}_0)$ of multivariate normal distributions with fixed covariance matrix $\boldsymbol{\Sigma}_0$ is already given in Example 2.18. Some other simple examples for EFs in canonical representations are shown in what follows, and the corresponding natural parameter spaces are determined.

Examples: $\mathfrak{poi}(\bullet)$, $\mathfrak{b}(n_0, \bullet)$, $\mathcal{N}(\bullet, \bullet)$, $\mathcal{G}(\bullet, \bullet)$

Example 2.37 Consider the representation of $\mathcal{P} = \mathfrak{poi}(\bullet)$ in Example 2.3 with $k = 1$, $Z_1(a) = \ln(a)$ for $a \in (0, \infty)$ and $T_1(x) = x$, $h(x) = 1/x!$ for $x \in \mathbb{N}_0$. Since

$$\int e^{\zeta x} \frac{1}{x!}\, d\mu_{\mathbb{N}_0}(x) = \sum_{x=0}^{\infty} e^{\zeta x} \frac{1}{x!} = \exp\left\{e^{\zeta}\right\}, \qquad \zeta \in \mathbb{R},$$

we have $\Xi^* = \mathbb{R} = Z_1((0, \infty))$. Hence, $\mathcal{P}$ is regular, and the canonical representation of $\mathcal{P}$ is given by the counting densities

$$f^*_{\zeta}(x) = C^*(\zeta)\, e^{\zeta x} \frac{1}{x!}, \qquad x \in \mathbb{N}_0,$$

with

$$C^*(\zeta) = \exp\left\{-e^{\zeta}\right\}$$

for $\zeta \in \mathbb{R}$.

Example 2.38 Consider the representation of $\mathcal{P} = \mathfrak{b}(n_0, \bullet)$ in Example 2.4 for fixed $n_0 \in \mathbb{N}$ with $k = 1$, $Z_1(p) = \ln(p/(1-p))$ for $p \in (0, 1)$ and $T_1(x) = x$, $h(x) = \binom{n_0}{x}$ for $x \in \{0, 1, \ldots, n_0\} = \mathcal{X}$. Since

$$\int e^{\zeta x} \binom{n_0}{x} d\mu_{\mathcal{X}}(x) = \sum_{x=0}^{n_0} e^{\zeta x} \binom{n_0}{x} = (1 + e^{\zeta})^{n_0}, \qquad \zeta \in \mathbb{R},$$

we have $\Xi^* = \mathbb{R} = Z_1((0, 1))$. Hence, $\mathcal{P}$ is regular, and the canonical representation of $\mathcal{P}$ is given by the counting densities

$$f_\zeta^*(x) = C^*(\zeta)\, e^{\zeta x} \binom{n_0}{x}, \qquad x \in \mathcal{X},$$

with

$$C^*(\zeta) = \left(1 + e^{\zeta}\right)^{-n_0}$$

for $\zeta \in \mathbb{R}$.

Example 2.39 Consider the representation of $\mathcal{P} = \mathcal{N}(\bullet, \bullet)$ in Example 2.10 with $k = 2$,

$$C(\mu, \sigma^2) = \frac{1}{\sqrt{\sigma^2}} \exp\left\{-\frac{\mu^2}{2\sigma^2}\right\},$$

$Z_1(\mu, \sigma^2) = \mu/\sigma^2$, and $Z_2(\mu, \sigma^2) = -1/(2\sigma^2)$ for $\mu \in \mathbb{R}$, $\sigma^2 \in (0, \infty)$, and $h(x) = 1/\sqrt{2\pi}$, $T_1(x) = x$, and $T_2(x) = x^2$ for $x \in \mathbb{R}$. Here, we have

$$\mathbb{R} \times (-\infty, 0) = \mathbf{Z}(\mathbb{R} \times (0, \infty)) \subset \Xi^*.$$

To establish that $\Xi^* = \mathbb{R} \times (-\infty, 0)$, it is sufficient to show that $(\zeta_1, 0)^t \notin \Xi^*$ for $\zeta_1 \in \mathbb{R}$, since Ξ^* is convex by Theorem 2.34. Indeed, for every $\zeta_1 \in \mathbb{R}$, we have

$$\int_{-\infty}^{\infty} e^{\zeta_1 x} \frac{1}{\sqrt{2\pi}}\, dx = \infty.$$

Hence, $\mathcal{P}$ is regular, and, by means of the parameter transformation

$$\left(\frac{\mu}{\sigma^2}, -\frac{1}{2\sigma^2}\right) = (\zeta_1, \zeta_2) \quad \Leftrightarrow \quad (\mu, \sigma^2) = \left(-\frac{\zeta_1}{2\zeta_2}, -\frac{1}{2\zeta_2}\right),$$

the canonical representation of $\mathcal{P}$ turns out to be

$$f^*_{\boldsymbol{\zeta}}(x) = C^*(\boldsymbol{\zeta})\, e^{\zeta_1 x + \zeta_2 x^2} \frac{1}{\sqrt{2\pi}}, \qquad x \in \mathbb{R},$$

with

$$C^*(\boldsymbol{\zeta}) = C\left(-\frac{\zeta_1}{2\zeta_2}, -\frac{1}{2\zeta_2}\right) = \sqrt{-2\zeta_2}\exp\left\{\frac{\zeta_1^2}{4\zeta_2}\right\}$$

for $\boldsymbol{\zeta} = (\zeta_1, \zeta_2)^t \in \mathbb{R} \times (-\infty, 0)$.

Example 2.40 Consider the representation of $\mathcal{P} = \mathcal{G}(\bullet, \bullet)$ in Example 2.12 with $k = 2$, $C(\alpha, \beta) = 1/[\Gamma(\beta)\alpha^\beta]$, $Z_1(\alpha, \beta) = -1/\alpha$, $Z_2(\alpha, \beta) = \beta$ for $\alpha, \beta \in (0, \infty)$, and $h(x) = 1/x$, $T_1(x) = x$, $T_2(x) = \ln(x)$ for $x \in (0, \infty)$. Here, we have

$$(-\infty, 0) \times (0, \infty) = \mathbf{Z}((0, \infty)^2) \subset \Xi^*.$$

To establish that $\Xi^* = (-\infty, 0) \times (0, \infty)$, it is sufficient to show that $(\zeta_1, 0)^t \notin \Xi^*$ and $(0, \zeta_2)^t \notin \Xi^*$ for $\zeta_1 \leq 0$ and $\zeta_2 > 0$, since Ξ^* is convex by Theorem 2.34. Indeed, for $\zeta_1 \leq 0$ and $\zeta_2 > 0$, we have

$$\int_0^\infty e^{\zeta_1 x} \frac{1}{x}\, dx \geq \int_0^1 e^{\zeta_1 x} \frac{1}{x}\, dx \geq e^{\zeta_1} \int_0^1 \frac{1}{x}\, dx = \infty$$

$$\text{and} \qquad \int_0^\infty e^{\zeta_2 \ln(x)} \frac{1}{x}\, dx = \frac{x^{\zeta_2}}{\zeta_2}\bigg|_0^\infty = \infty.$$

Hence, $\mathcal{P}$ is regular, and, by means of the parameter transformation $\zeta_1 = -1/\alpha$ and $\zeta_2 = \beta$, the canonical representation of $\mathcal{P}$ turns out to be

$$f^*_{\boldsymbol{\zeta}}(x) = C^*(\boldsymbol{\zeta})\, e^{\zeta_1 x + \zeta_2 \ln(x)} \frac{1}{x}, \qquad x \in (0, \infty),$$

with

$$C^*(\zeta) = C\left(-\frac{1}{\zeta_1}, \zeta_2\right) = \frac{(-\zeta_1)^{\zeta_2}}{\Gamma(\zeta_2)}$$

for $\boldsymbol{\zeta} = (\zeta_1, \zeta_2)^t \in (-\infty, 0) \times (0, \infty)$.

The EFs considered in the preceding examples are all full and moreover regular, since the natural parameter space turns out to be open. Indeed, this is the case for most of the common EFs. An example for a full but non-regular EF is provided by the full family of inverse normal distributions (see, e.g., [4, p. 117] or [20, p. 72]).

Example: $\mathcal{IN}(\bullet, \bullet)$

Example 2.41 Consider the representation of $\mathcal{P} = \mathcal{IN}(\bullet, \bullet)$ in Example 2.11 with $k = 2$,

$$C(\mu, \eta) = \sqrt{\eta} \exp\left\{\frac{\eta}{\mu}\right\},$$

$Z_1(\mu, \eta) = -\eta/(2\mu^2)$, and $Z_2(\mu, \eta) = -\eta/2$ for $\mu, \eta \in (0, \infty)$, and $h(x) = \sqrt{1/(2\pi x^3)}$, $T_1(x) = x$, and $T_2(x) = 1/x$ for $x \in (0, \infty)$. Here, we have

$$(-\infty, 0)^2 = \mathbf{Z}((0, \infty)^2) \subset \Xi^*.$$

However, it turns out that $\Xi^* = (-\infty, 0] \times (-\infty, 0)$, which can be seen as follows.

First, we have $(0, \zeta_2)^t \in \Xi^*$ for $\zeta_2 < 0$, since by substituting $z = 1/x$

$$\int_0^\infty e^{\zeta_2/x} \sqrt{\frac{1}{2\pi x^3}}\, dx = \sqrt{\frac{1}{2\pi}} \int_0^\infty e^{\zeta_2 z} z^{-1/2}\, dz$$

$$= \sqrt{\frac{1}{2\pi}} \frac{\Gamma(1/2)}{(-\zeta_2)^{1/2}} = \sqrt{\frac{1}{-2\zeta_2}} < \infty.$$

Moreover, it holds that $(\zeta_1, 0)^t \notin \Xi^*$ for $\zeta_1 \le 0$, since

$$\int_0^\infty e^{\zeta_1 x}\sqrt{\frac{1}{2\pi x^3}}\,dx \ge \sqrt{\frac{1}{2\pi}}\int_0^1 e^{\zeta_1 x}\sqrt{\frac{1}{x^3}}\,dx$$
$$\ge \sqrt{\frac{1}{2\pi}}e^{\zeta_1}\int_0^1 \frac{1}{x}\,dx = \infty\,.$$

Finally, we have $(\zeta_1, \zeta_2)^t \notin \Xi^*$ for $\zeta_1 > 0$ and $\zeta_2 < 0$, since by using the series representation of $\exp\{\zeta_1 x\}$

$$\int_0^\infty e^{\zeta_1 x+\zeta_2/x}\sqrt{\frac{1}{2\pi x^3}}\,dx \ge \sqrt{\frac{1}{2\pi}}\int_1^\infty e^{\zeta_1 x+\zeta_2/x}\sqrt{\frac{1}{x^3}}\,dx$$
$$\ge \sqrt{\frac{1}{2\pi}}e^{\zeta_2}\int_1^\infty e^{\zeta_1 x}\frac{1}{x^2}\,dx$$
$$\ge \sqrt{\frac{1}{2\pi}}e^{\zeta_2}\int_1^\infty \frac{(\zeta_1 x)^2}{2!}\frac{1}{x^2}\,dx = \infty\,.$$

The convexity of Ξ^* as pointed out in Theorem 2.34 now ensures that $\Xi^* = (-\infty, 0] \times (-\infty, 0)$. In particular, $\mathcal{P}$ is not full. By using the parameter transformation

$$\left(-\frac{\eta}{2\mu^2}, -\frac{\eta}{2}\right) = (\zeta_1, \zeta_2) \quad\Leftrightarrow\quad (\mu, \eta) = \left(\sqrt{\frac{\zeta_2}{\zeta_1}}, -2\zeta_2\right)$$

the canonical representation of $\mathcal{P}$ is given by

$$f_{\boldsymbol{\zeta}}^*(x) = C^*(\boldsymbol{\zeta})\,e^{\zeta_1 x+\zeta_2/x}\sqrt{\frac{1}{2\pi x^3}}\,,\qquad x \in (0, \infty)\,,$$

with

$$C^*(\boldsymbol{\zeta}) = C\left(\sqrt{\frac{\zeta_2}{\zeta_1}}, -2\zeta_2\right) = \sqrt{-2\zeta_2}\,e^{2\sqrt{\zeta_1\zeta_2}}$$

for $\boldsymbol{\zeta} = (\zeta_1, \zeta_2)^t \in (-\infty, 0)^2$. Note that the associated full EF $\{P_{\boldsymbol{\zeta}}^* : \boldsymbol{\zeta} \in (-\infty, 0] \times (-\infty, 0)\}$ with $C^*(0, \zeta_2) = \sqrt{-2\zeta_2}$ for $\zeta_2 < 0$ is not regular.

Having seen that the natural parameter space of the EF is not open in general, we address a simple sufficient condition in the following lemma guaranteeing that it has at least some inner points. The proof makes use of the convexity property of Ξ^* and Lemma 2.22 (for details, see [63, p. 150]).

Lemma 2.42 *Let $\mathcal{P}$ be an EF with representation (2.1). If $Z_1, \ldots, Z_k$ are affinely independent, then $int(\Xi^*) \neq \emptyset$.*

To address further properties related to the natural parametrization, we introduce a function, which is of high relevance in statistical inference.

Definition 2.43 Let $\mathcal{P}$ be an EF with canonical representation (2.6). The mapping $\kappa : \Xi \to \mathbb{R}$ defined by $\kappa = -\ln(C^*)$ is called the *cumulant function* of $\mathcal{P}$.

For the motivation of the term cumulant function in Definition 2.43 and for remarks on so-called cumulants, we refer to Sects. 2.4 and 3.1.

The following properties of the cumulant function are immediately obtained from the proof of Theorem 2.34 and Lemma 2.30.

Theorem 2.44 *Let $\mathcal{P}$ be a full EF with canonical representation (2.6) and cumulant function $\kappa = -\ln(C^*)$ defined on Ξ^*. Then, we have:*

(a) κ is convex, i.e., if $\boldsymbol{\zeta}, \boldsymbol{\eta} \in \Xi^*$ and $\alpha \in (0, 1)$, then

$$\kappa(\alpha\boldsymbol{\zeta} + (1-\alpha)\boldsymbol{\eta}) \leq \alpha\kappa(\boldsymbol{\zeta}) + (1-\alpha)\kappa(\boldsymbol{\eta}) . \tag{2.8}$$

Here, equality holds true if and only if $P^*_{\boldsymbol{\zeta}} = P^*_{\boldsymbol{\eta}}$.

(b) If $T_1, \ldots, T_k$ are ν-affinely independent, then κ is strictly convex on Ξ^*, i.e., equality in Eq. (2.8) holds true if and only if $\boldsymbol{\zeta} = \boldsymbol{\eta}$.

Note that, since κ is convex and finite on Ξ^*, it is continuous on the interior $int(\Xi^*)$ of Ξ^* (see, e.g., [51, Section 10]). For maximum likelihood estimation in a subsequent section, it will be convenient to extend κ in a natural way to a function on $\mathbb{R}^k$. The following property then directly follows from Fatou's lemma (see [20, pp. 19/20]). Fatou's lemma along with its proof can be found, e.g., in [17, p. 209].

Lemma 2.45 *Let $\mathcal{P}$ be a full EF with canonical representation (2.6) and cumulant function $\kappa = -\ln(C^*)$ on Ξ^*. Moreover, let $\tilde{\kappa} : \mathbb{R}^k \to \mathbb{R} \cup \{\infty\}$ be the extension of κ defined by $\tilde{\kappa}(\boldsymbol{\zeta}) = \infty$ for $\boldsymbol{\zeta} \in \mathbb{R}^k \setminus \Xi^*$. Then, $\tilde{\kappa}$ is lower semi-continuous, i.e.,*

$$\liminf_{\boldsymbol{\eta} \to \boldsymbol{\zeta}} \tilde{\kappa}(\boldsymbol{\eta}) \geq \tilde{\kappa}(\boldsymbol{\zeta}) \quad \text{for every } \boldsymbol{\zeta} \in \mathbb{R}^k .$$

Moreover, $\tilde{\kappa}$ is continuous on $int(\Xi^*)$.

When aiming for inference with a given EF, it is advisable to find a minimal representation, first, before transforming it to a canonical representation. Otherwise, statistical problems may arise as it is demonstrated in the following example, where we discuss the structure of the multinomial EF (see [20, pp. 4–6]).

Example: $\mathfrak{m}(n_0, \bullet)$

Example 2.46 Consider the representation of $\mathcal{P} = \mathfrak{m}(n_0, \bullet)$ in Example 2.8 for fixed $n_0 \in \mathbb{N}$ with $C(\boldsymbol{p}) = 1$,

$$Z_j(\boldsymbol{p}) = \ln(p_j), \quad \boldsymbol{p} \in \Theta = \{(q_1, \ldots, q_k)^t \in (0,1)^k : \sum_{i=1}^k q_i = 1\},$$

and $h(\boldsymbol{x}) = n_0!/\prod_{i=1}^k x_i!$,

$$T_j(\boldsymbol{x}) = x_j, \quad \boldsymbol{x} \in \mathcal{X} = \{(y_1, \ldots, y_k)^t \in \mathbb{N}_0^k : \sum_{i=1}^k y_i = n_0\},$$

for $j \in \{1, \ldots, k\}$. For $\boldsymbol{\zeta} = (\zeta_1, \ldots, \zeta_k)^t \in \mathbb{R}^k$, it follows by the multinomial theorem that

$$\begin{aligned}\int \exp\left\{\sum_{j=1}^k \zeta_j x_j\right\} h(\boldsymbol{x})\, d\mu_{\mathcal{X}}(\boldsymbol{x}) &= \sum_{\boldsymbol{x}\in\mathcal{X}} \frac{n_0!}{\prod_{i=1}^k x_i!} \prod_{j=1}^k (e^{\zeta_j})^{x_j} \\ &= \left(\sum_{j=1}^k e^{\zeta_j}\right)^{n_0}.\end{aligned}$$

Hence, we have $\Xi^* = \mathbb{R}^k$, and, since $\boldsymbol{Z}(\Theta) \subset (-\infty, 0)^k$, $\mathcal{P}$ is not full. The full EF is given by $\mathcal{P}^* = \{P_{\boldsymbol{\zeta}}^* : \boldsymbol{\zeta} \in \mathbb{R}^k\}$, where $P_{\boldsymbol{\zeta}}^*$ has counting density

$$f_{\boldsymbol{\zeta}}^*(\boldsymbol{x}) = \left(\sum_{j=1}^k e^{\zeta_j}\right)^{-n_0} \exp\left\{\sum_{j=1}^k \zeta_j x_j\right\} h(\boldsymbol{x}), \qquad \boldsymbol{x} \in \mathcal{X},$$

for $\boldsymbol{\zeta} \in \mathbb{R}^k$. Nevertheless, it holds that $\mathcal{P} = \mathcal{P}^*$, which can be seen as follows. First, for $\boldsymbol{\zeta} \in \mathbb{R}^k$, $\boldsymbol{1}^{(k)} = (1, \ldots, 1)^t \in \mathbb{R}^k$, and $a \in \mathbb{R}$, we have

$$f_{\boldsymbol{\zeta}+a\boldsymbol{1}^{(k)}}^*(\boldsymbol{x}) = \left(\sum_{j=1}^k e^{\zeta_j + a}\right)^{-n_0} \exp\left\{\sum_{j=1}^k (\zeta_j + a)\, x_j\right\} h(\boldsymbol{x})$$

$$= e^{-n_0 a} \exp\left\{a \sum_{j=1}^{k} x_j\right\} f_{\boldsymbol{\zeta}}^*(\boldsymbol{x})$$

$$= f_{\boldsymbol{\zeta}}^*(\boldsymbol{x}), \qquad \boldsymbol{x} \in \mathcal{X}.$$

Hence, $P_{\boldsymbol{\zeta}}^* = P_{\boldsymbol{\zeta}+a\mathbf{1}^{(k)}}^*$. Now, let $\boldsymbol{\zeta} \in \mathbb{R}^k$. We have to show that there exists some $\boldsymbol{p} \in \Theta$ with $\mathfrak{m}(n_0, \boldsymbol{p}) = P_{\boldsymbol{\zeta}}^*$. To this end, let $\boldsymbol{p} = (p_1, \ldots, p_k)^t$ with

$$p_i = \exp\left\{\zeta_i - \ln\left(\sum_{j=1}^{k} e^{\zeta_j}\right)\right\}, \quad 1 \le i \le k.$$

Obviously, $p_i > 0$ for $1 \le i \le k$, and $\sum_{j=1}^{k} p_j = 1$, such that $\boldsymbol{p} \in \Theta$. Moreover, since $f_{n_0,\boldsymbol{p}} = f_{\boldsymbol{Z}(\boldsymbol{p})}^*$ by definition, it follows for $a = -\ln(\sum_{j=1}^{k} \exp\{\zeta_j\})$ that

$$\mathfrak{m}(n_0, \boldsymbol{p}) = P_{\boldsymbol{Z}(\boldsymbol{p})}^* = P_{\boldsymbol{\zeta}+a\mathbf{1}^{(k)}}^* = P_{\boldsymbol{\zeta}}^*.$$

Hence, $\mathcal{P} = \mathcal{P}^*$ is shown. In particular, this yields that the parameter $\boldsymbol{\zeta} \in \Xi^*$ is not identifiable.

This problem occurs, since the representation of $\mathcal{P}$ in Example 2.8 is not minimal. Indeed, we have $ord(\mathcal{P}) = k - 1$, which is shown in the following. First, we rewrite

$$f_{n_0,\boldsymbol{p}}(\boldsymbol{x}) = \exp\left\{\sum_{j=1}^{k-1} \ln(p_j)\, x_j + \ln(p_k)\left(n_0 - \sum_{j=1}^{k-1} x_j\right)\right\} h(\boldsymbol{x})$$

$$= p_k^{n_0} \exp\left\{\sum_{j=1}^{k-1} (\ln(p_j) - \ln(p_k)) x_j\right\} h(\boldsymbol{x}), \qquad \boldsymbol{x} \in \mathcal{X}. \quad (2.9)$$

This is another representation of $\mathcal{P}$ with parameter functions $\tilde{Z}_j(\boldsymbol{p}) = \ln(p_j) - \ln(p_k)$ for $\boldsymbol{p} \in \Theta$ and statistics $T_j(\boldsymbol{x}) = x_j$ for $\boldsymbol{x} \in \mathcal{X}$, $1 \le j \le k - 1$. Hence,

$ord(\mathcal{P}) \leq k-1$. Since $\emptyset$ is the only set $N \subset \mathcal{X}$ with $\nu(N) = 0$, we show that $T_1, \ldots, T_{k-1}$ are affinely independent. Let $a_0, a_1, \ldots, a_{k-1} \in \mathbb{R}$ with

$$0 = a_0 + \sum_{j=1}^{k-1} a_j T_j(\boldsymbol{x}) = a_0 + \sum_{j=1}^{k-1} a_j x_j \qquad \text{for all } \boldsymbol{x} \in \mathcal{X}. \tag{2.10}$$

Moreover, we denote by $\boldsymbol{e}_j^{(k)}$ the j-th unit vector in $\mathbb{R}^k$. Then, setting $\boldsymbol{x} = n_0 \boldsymbol{e}_k^{(k)} \in \mathcal{X}$ in Eq. (2.10) gives $a_0 = 0$, and the choice $\boldsymbol{x} = n_0 \boldsymbol{e}_j^{(k)} \in \mathcal{X}$ leads to $a_j = 0$, $1 \leq j \leq k-1$. To show that $\tilde{Z}_1, \ldots, \tilde{Z}_{k-1}$ are affinely independent, let $\boldsymbol{p}^{(0)} = \mathbf{1}^{(k)}/k \in \Theta$ and $\boldsymbol{p}^{(j)} = (\mathbf{1}^{(k)} + \boldsymbol{e}_j^{(k)})/(k+1) \in \Theta$, $1 \leq j \leq k-1$. By setting $\tilde{\boldsymbol{Z}} = (\tilde{Z}_1, \ldots, \tilde{Z}_{k-1})^t$, we have

$$\tilde{\boldsymbol{Z}}(\boldsymbol{p}^{(j)}) - \tilde{\boldsymbol{Z}}(\boldsymbol{p}^{(0)}) = \tilde{\boldsymbol{Z}}(\boldsymbol{p}^{(j)}) = \ln(2)\, \boldsymbol{e}_j^{(k-1)} \in \mathbb{R}^{k-1}, \quad 1 \leq j \leq k-1.$$

From Lemma 2.22, we obtain that $\tilde{Z}_1, \ldots, \tilde{Z}_{k-1}$ are affinely independent, and applying Theorem 2.23 gives $ord(\mathcal{P}) = k-1$. In particular, representation (2.9) is minimal. Now, by using the multinomial theorem again, $\Xi^* = \mathbb{R}^{k-1} = \tilde{\boldsymbol{Z}}(\Theta)$, such that $\mathcal{P}$ is full and regular. Finally, by setting $\zeta_j = \ln(p_j) - \ln(p_k)$, $1 \leq j \leq k-1$, in density (2.9) and by noticing that then

$$p_k = 1 - \sum_{j=1}^{k-1} p_j = 1 - p_k \sum_{j=1}^{k-1} e^{\zeta_j} \quad \text{and thus} \quad p_k = \left(1 + \sum_{j=1}^{k-1} e^{\zeta_j}\right)^{-1},$$

a minimal canonical representation of $\mathcal{P}$ is given by the counting densities

$$\tilde{f}_{\boldsymbol{\zeta}}^*(\boldsymbol{x}) = \left(1 + \sum_{j=1}^{k-1} e^{\zeta_j}\right)^{-n_0} \exp\left\{\sum_{j=1}^{k-1} \zeta_j x_j\right\} h(\boldsymbol{x}), \qquad \boldsymbol{x} \in \mathcal{X},$$

for $\boldsymbol{\zeta} \in \mathbb{R}^{k-1}$.

2.4 Analytical Properties and Mean Value Parametrization

We now turn to useful analytical properties of the EF in natural parametrization. Essentially, they are consequences of the following lemma, which can be shown by using the Lebesgue dominated-convergence theorem; a detailed proof is provided, e.g., in [40, pp. 49/50].

Lemma 2.47 *Let $\mathcal{P}$ be an EF with canonical representation (2.6), and let $A \subset \Xi$ be an open set. Moreover, let the function $\varphi : (\mathcal{X}, \mathcal{B}) \to (\mathbb{R}^1, \mathbb{B}^1)$ be $P_{\boldsymbol{\zeta}}^*$-integrable for all $\boldsymbol{\zeta} = (\zeta_1, \dots, \zeta_k)^t \in A$. Then, the function $\delta : A \to \mathbb{R}$ defined by*

$$\delta(\boldsymbol{\zeta}) = \int \varphi(x) \exp\left\{\sum_{j=1}^{k} \zeta_j T_j(x)\right\} h(x)\, d\mu(x), \qquad \boldsymbol{\zeta} \in A,$$

is infinitely often differentiable, and the partial derivatives can be obtained by differentiating under the integral sign, i.e.,

$$\frac{\partial^{l_1}}{\partial \zeta_1^{l_1}} \cdots \frac{\partial^{l_k}}{\partial \zeta_k^{l_k}} \delta(\boldsymbol{\zeta}) = \int \varphi(x)\, T_1^{l_1}(x) \dots T_k^{l_k}(x) \exp\left\{\sum_{j=1}^{k} \zeta_j T_j(x)\right\} h(x)\, d\mu(x) \tag{2.11}$$

for $\boldsymbol{\zeta} \in A$ and $l_1, \dots, l_k \in \mathbb{N}_0$.

Remark 2.48 Lemma 2.47 can be extended to functions δ with complex arguments: If δ is defined on the complex set $\{z = \boldsymbol{\zeta} + i\boldsymbol{\eta} \in \mathbb{C}^k : \boldsymbol{\zeta} \in A\}$, then δ is a holomorphic function of every variable z_j for fixed other components z_i, $i \neq j$. As in Lemma 2.47, its (complex) derivatives can be obtained by differentiating under the integral sign. For a proof, see, e.g., [40, pp. 49/50].

The usefulness of Lemma 2.47 is that it yields existence and simple representations for the moments of $\boldsymbol{T}$. Setting $\varphi \equiv 1$, which is $P_{\boldsymbol{\zeta}}^*$-integrable for all $\boldsymbol{\zeta} \in \Xi^*$ as a constant function, and multiplying both sides of Eq. (2.11) by $C^*(\boldsymbol{\zeta})$, we directly obtain the following theorem by noticing that $E_{\boldsymbol{\zeta}}[T_1^{l_1} \dots T_k^{l_k}] = \int T_1^{l_1} \dots T_k^{l_k} f_{\boldsymbol{\zeta}}^* d\mu$.

Theorem 2.49 *Let $\mathcal{P}$ be an EF with canonical representation (2.6). Then, for $\boldsymbol{\zeta} \in int(\Xi)$, $\boldsymbol{T} = (T_1, \dots, T_k)^t$ has finite multivariate moments of any order with respect to $P_{\boldsymbol{\zeta}}^*$, which are given by*

$$E_{\boldsymbol{\zeta}}[T_1^{l_1} \dots T_k^{l_k}] = C^*(\boldsymbol{\zeta}) \frac{\partial^{l_1}}{\partial \zeta_1^{l_1}} \cdots \frac{\partial^{l_k}}{\partial \zeta_k^{l_k}} \int \exp\left\{\sum_{j=1}^{k} \zeta_j T_j\right\} h\, d\mu$$

for $l_1, \dots, l_k \in \mathbb{N}_0$.

As another important finding, the mean and covariance matrix of $\boldsymbol{T}$ can be obtained as derivatives of the cumulant function $\kappa = -\ln(C^*)$ introduced in Definition 2.43; the proof gives insight into the convenient structure of the canonical representation.

Corollary 2.50 *Let $\mathcal{P}$ be an EF with canonical representation (2.6). Then, the functions C^* and $\kappa = -\ln(C^*)$ are infinitely often differentiable at every $\boldsymbol{\zeta} \in int(\Xi)$, where*

$$\nabla\kappa(\boldsymbol{\zeta}) = E_{\boldsymbol{\zeta}}[\boldsymbol{T}],$$

$$\mathbf{H}_{\kappa}(\boldsymbol{\zeta}) = \mathbf{Cov}_{\boldsymbol{\zeta}}(\boldsymbol{T}).$$

Here, $\nabla\kappa(\boldsymbol{\zeta})$ and $\mathbf{H}_{\kappa}(\boldsymbol{\zeta})$ denote the gradient and the Hessian matrix of κ evaluated at $\boldsymbol{\zeta}$.

Proof By Lemma 2.47 with $\varphi \equiv 1$, the function $1/C^*$ and thus C^* and $\kappa = -\ln(C^*)$ are infinitely often differentiable at $\boldsymbol{\zeta} \in int(\Xi)$. Moreover, with $\nu = h\mu$, we obtain that

$$\frac{\partial}{\partial \zeta_i}\kappa(\boldsymbol{\zeta}) = \frac{\partial}{\partial \zeta_i}\ln\left(\int e^{\boldsymbol{\zeta}^t\boldsymbol{T}}\,d\nu\right) = \frac{\int T_i e^{\boldsymbol{\zeta}^t\boldsymbol{T}}\,d\nu}{\int e^{\boldsymbol{\zeta}^t\boldsymbol{T}}\,d\nu} = E_{\boldsymbol{\zeta}}[T_i]$$

for $1 \le i \le k$. Applying Lemma 2.47 with $\varphi = T_i$, which is admissible by Theorem 2.49, then yields

$$\begin{aligned}\frac{\partial^2}{\partial \zeta_i\,\partial \zeta_j}\kappa(\boldsymbol{\zeta}) &= \frac{\partial}{\partial \zeta_j}\left(\frac{\int T_i e^{\boldsymbol{\zeta}^t\boldsymbol{T}}\,d\nu}{\int e^{\boldsymbol{\zeta}^t\boldsymbol{T}}\,d\nu}\right)\\ &= \frac{(\int T_iT_j e^{\boldsymbol{\zeta}^t\boldsymbol{T}}\,d\nu)(\int e^{\boldsymbol{\zeta}^t\boldsymbol{T}}\,d\nu) - (\int T_i e^{\boldsymbol{\zeta}^t\boldsymbol{T}}\,d\nu)(\int T_j e^{\boldsymbol{\zeta}^t\boldsymbol{T}}\,d\nu)}{(\int e^{\boldsymbol{\zeta}^t\boldsymbol{T}}\,d\nu)^2}\\ &= E_{\boldsymbol{\zeta}}[T_iT_j] - E_{\boldsymbol{\zeta}}[T_i]E_{\boldsymbol{\zeta}}[T_j] = \mathrm{Cov}_{\boldsymbol{\zeta}}(T_i, T_j)\end{aligned}$$

for $1 \le i, j \le k$. □

Moments in EFs with canonical representation are easily determined by the respective normalizing constant $C^*(\boldsymbol{\zeta})$.

Examples: $\mathfrak{nb}(r_0,\bullet)$, $\mathcal{N}(\bullet,\bullet)$, $\mathcal{G}(\bullet,\bullet)$, $\mathcal{N}_k(\bullet,\boldsymbol{\Sigma}_0)$

Example 2.51 From Example 2.5, it is readily seen that the EF $\mathcal{P} = \mathfrak{nb}(r_0,\bullet)$ is regular with canonical representation

$$f_{\zeta}^*(x) = C^*(\zeta)\,e^{\zeta x}\binom{x+r_0-1}{x}, \qquad x \in \mathbb{N}_0,$$

with $C^*(\zeta) = (1 - \exp\{\zeta\})^{r_0}$ for $\zeta \in \Xi^* = (-\infty, 0)$. Hence,

$$\kappa(\zeta) = -r_0 \ln\left(1 - e^{\zeta}\right), \qquad \zeta \in (-\infty, 0),$$

and, by using Corollary 2.50, the mean and variance of the negative binomial distribution P_ζ^* are given by

$$\kappa'(\zeta) = \frac{r_0 \exp\{\zeta\}}{1 - \exp\{\zeta\}} \quad \text{and} \quad \kappa''(\zeta) = \frac{r_0 \exp\{\zeta\}}{(1 - \exp\{\zeta\})^2}.$$

In the original parametrization, this yields the expressions $r_0(1-p)/p$ and $r_0(1-p)/p^2$ for the mean and variance of $P_p = \mathfrak{nb}(r_0, p)$.

Example 2.52 In Example 2.39, the canonical representation of $\mathcal{P} = \mathcal{N}(\bullet, \bullet)$ yields

$$C^*(\boldsymbol{\zeta}) = \sqrt{-2\zeta_2} \exp\left\{\frac{\zeta_1^2}{4\zeta_2}\right\}, \qquad \boldsymbol{\zeta} = (\zeta_1, \zeta_2)^t \in \mathbb{R} \times (-\infty, 0),$$

and $\boldsymbol{T}(x) = (T_1(x), T_2(x))^t = (x, x^2)^t$, $x \in \mathbb{R}$. Hence, by Corollary 2.50 with $\kappa(\boldsymbol{\zeta}) = -\ln(-2\zeta_2)/2 - \zeta_1^2/(4\zeta_2)$,

$$E_{\boldsymbol{\zeta}}[T_1] = \frac{\partial}{\partial \zeta_1}\kappa(\boldsymbol{\zeta}) = -\frac{\zeta_1}{2\zeta_2}$$

$$\text{and} \quad E_{\boldsymbol{\zeta}}[T_2] = \frac{\partial}{\partial \zeta_2}\kappa(\boldsymbol{\zeta}) = -\frac{1}{2\zeta_2} + \frac{\zeta_1^2}{4\zeta_2^2}$$

for $\boldsymbol{\zeta} = (\zeta_1, \zeta_2)^t \in \mathbb{R} \times (-\infty, 0)$. In terms of the common parametrization of the univariate normal distribution (see Example 2.10), we find for a random variable $X \sim \mathcal{N}(\mu, \sigma^2)$ with parameters $(\mu, \sigma^2) = (-\zeta_1/(2\zeta_2), -1/(2\zeta_2))^t$ that the means of $X = T_1(X)$ and $X^2 = T_2(X)$ are given by μ and $\sigma^2 + \mu^2$; the variance of X is then equal to σ^2.

Example 2.53 For $\mathcal{P} = \mathcal{G}(\bullet, \bullet)$, we conclude from Example 2.40 that

$$\kappa(\boldsymbol{\zeta}) = \ln(\Gamma(\zeta_2)) - \zeta_2 \ln(-\zeta_1), \qquad \boldsymbol{\zeta} = (\zeta_1, \zeta_2)^t \in (-\infty, 0) \times (0, \infty).$$

Hence, by using Corollary 2.50, we have for $\boldsymbol{T}(x) = (x, \ln(x))^t$, $x \in (0, \infty)$, that

$$E_{\boldsymbol{\zeta}}[\boldsymbol{T}] = \nabla\kappa(\boldsymbol{\zeta}) = \left(-\frac{\zeta_2}{\zeta_1}, \psi(\zeta_2) - \ln(-\zeta_1)\right)^t, \qquad \boldsymbol{\zeta} \in (-\infty, 0) \times (0, \infty),$$

where $\psi(y) = [\ln(\Gamma(y))]' = \Gamma'(y)/\Gamma(y)$, $y \in (0, \infty)$, denotes the digamma function (see [22, p. 258]). Moreover, it follows that

$$\mathbf{Cov}_{\boldsymbol{\zeta}}(\boldsymbol{T}) = \mathbf{H}_\kappa(\boldsymbol{\zeta}) = \begin{pmatrix} \frac{\zeta_2}{\zeta_1^2} & -\frac{1}{\zeta_1} \\ -\frac{1}{\zeta_1} & \psi_1(\zeta_2) \end{pmatrix}, \qquad \boldsymbol{\zeta} \in (-\infty, 0) \times (0, \infty),$$

where $\psi_1 = \psi'$ denotes the trigamma function (see [22, p. 260]). In particular, the mean and variance of the gamma distribution $P_{\boldsymbol{\zeta}}^*$ are given by $-\zeta_2/\zeta_1$ and ζ_2/ζ_1^2.

Example 2.54 For the EF $\mathcal{P} = \mathcal{N}_k(\bullet, \boldsymbol{\Sigma}_0)$ of multivariate normal distributions as in Example 2.18, which is already given in natural parametrization ($\boldsymbol{\zeta} = \boldsymbol{\mu}$, $C^* = C$), we have

$$C(\boldsymbol{\mu}) = \exp\left\{-\frac{||\boldsymbol{\mu}||_{\boldsymbol{\Sigma}_0}^2}{2}\right\} = \exp\left\{-\frac{1}{2}\boldsymbol{\mu}^t \boldsymbol{\Sigma}_0^{-1} \boldsymbol{\mu}\right\}, \qquad \boldsymbol{\mu} \in \mathbb{R}^k.$$

Then, by Corollary 2.50 with $\kappa(\boldsymbol{\mu}) = \boldsymbol{\mu}^t \boldsymbol{\Sigma}_0^{-1} \boldsymbol{\mu}/2$,

$$E_{\boldsymbol{\mu}}[\boldsymbol{T}] = \nabla\kappa(\boldsymbol{\mu}) = \boldsymbol{\Sigma}_0^{-1}\boldsymbol{\mu},$$

$$\mathbf{Cov}_{\boldsymbol{\mu}}(\boldsymbol{T}) = \mathbf{H}_\kappa(\boldsymbol{\mu}) = \boldsymbol{\Sigma}_0^{-1}, \qquad \boldsymbol{\mu} \in \mathbb{R}^k,$$

where $\boldsymbol{T}(\boldsymbol{x}) = \boldsymbol{\Sigma}_0^{-1}\boldsymbol{x}$, $\boldsymbol{x} \in \mathbb{R}^k$. Hence, for a random vector $\boldsymbol{X} \sim \mathcal{N}_k(\boldsymbol{\mu}, \boldsymbol{\Sigma}_0)$, we find with the identity $\boldsymbol{X} = \boldsymbol{\Sigma}_0 \boldsymbol{T}(\boldsymbol{X})$ that the mean and covariance matrix of $\boldsymbol{X}$ are given by $\boldsymbol{\Sigma}_0 E_{\boldsymbol{\mu}}[\boldsymbol{T}] = \boldsymbol{\mu}$ and $\boldsymbol{\Sigma}_0 \mathbf{Cov}_{\boldsymbol{\mu}}(\boldsymbol{T})\boldsymbol{\Sigma}_0 = \boldsymbol{\Sigma}_0$.

Lemma 2.47 and Corollary 2.50 may be applied to establish the following result. It is important for the derivation of optimal statistical tests.

Corollary 2.55 *Under the assumptions of Lemma 2.47, the mapping*

$$\beta_\varphi : \quad A \to \mathbb{R} : \quad \boldsymbol{\zeta} \mapsto E_{\boldsymbol{\zeta}}[\varphi]$$

is infinitely often differentiable with gradient

$$\nabla\beta_\varphi(\boldsymbol{\zeta}) = E_{\boldsymbol{\zeta}}[\varphi\,\boldsymbol{T}] - E_{\boldsymbol{\zeta}}[\varphi]\,E_{\boldsymbol{\zeta}}[\boldsymbol{T}] = \mathbf{Cov}_{\boldsymbol{\zeta}}(\varphi, \boldsymbol{T}), \qquad \boldsymbol{\zeta} \in A.$$

Proof Since

$$\beta_\varphi(\boldsymbol{\zeta}) = C^*(\boldsymbol{\zeta}) \int \varphi\, e^{\boldsymbol{\zeta}^t \boldsymbol{T}}\, h\, d\mu\,, \qquad \boldsymbol{\zeta} \in A\,,$$

β_φ is infinitely often differentiable by Lemma 2.47 and Corollary 2.50. Moreover, for $1 \le i \le k$, we obtain that

$$\frac{\partial}{\partial \zeta_i} C^*(\boldsymbol{\zeta}) = \frac{\partial}{\partial \zeta_i}\left[\left(\int e^{\boldsymbol{\zeta}^t \boldsymbol{T}}\, h\, d\mu\right)^{-1}\right] = -\frac{\int T_i\, e^{\boldsymbol{\zeta}^t \boldsymbol{T}}\, h\, d\mu}{(\int e^{\boldsymbol{\zeta}^t \boldsymbol{T}}\, h\, d\mu)^2} = -\,C^*(\boldsymbol{\zeta})\, E_{\boldsymbol{\zeta}}[T_i]$$

and, hence,

$$\begin{aligned}\frac{\partial}{\partial \zeta_i}\beta_\varphi(\boldsymbol{\zeta}) &= \left(\frac{\partial}{\partial \zeta_i} C^*(\boldsymbol{\zeta})\right) \int \varphi\, e^{\boldsymbol{\zeta}^t \boldsymbol{T}}\, h\, d\mu + C^*(\boldsymbol{\zeta}) \int \varphi\, T_i\, e^{\boldsymbol{\zeta}^t \boldsymbol{T}}\, h\, d\mu \\ &= E_{\boldsymbol{\zeta}}[\varphi\, T_i] - E_{\boldsymbol{\zeta}}[\varphi]\, E_{\boldsymbol{\zeta}}[T_i]\,.\end{aligned}$$

□

There is an important function, which describes the relationship between the natural parameter space Ξ^* and the expectation space of the vector $\boldsymbol{T}$ of statistics. Its properties allow for another parametrization of a regular EF, and they are also useful in point estimation.

Theorem 2.56 *Let $\mathcal{P}$ be a full EF with minimal canonical representation (2.6). Then, the so-called mean value function*

$$\pi: \quad int(\Xi^*) \to \pi(int(\Xi^*)): \quad \boldsymbol{\zeta} \mapsto E_{\boldsymbol{\zeta}}[\boldsymbol{T}]$$

has the following properties:

(a) $\pi(\boldsymbol{\zeta}) = \nabla\kappa(\boldsymbol{\zeta})$ for every $\boldsymbol{\zeta} \in int(\Xi^*)$.
(b) π is continuously differentiable with Jacobian matrix

$$\mathbf{D}_\pi(\boldsymbol{\zeta}) = \mathbf{H}_\kappa(\boldsymbol{\zeta}) = \mathbf{Cov}_{\boldsymbol{\zeta}}(\boldsymbol{T}) > 0\,, \qquad \boldsymbol{\zeta} \in int(\Xi^*)\,.$$

(c) π is bijective and has a continuously differentiable inverse function π^{-1} : $\pi(int(\Xi^*)) \to int(\Xi^*)$.

Proof Assertions (a) and (b) directly follow from Corollary 2.50 together with Theorem 2.23 and Lemma 2.26. For statement (c), let $\boldsymbol{\zeta}, \boldsymbol{\eta} \in int(\Xi^*)$ with $\boldsymbol{\zeta} \ne \boldsymbol{\eta}$. By Theorem 2.23 and 2.44(b), κ is strictly convex on Ξ^*. Hence, by using part (a),

$$(\boldsymbol{\eta} - \boldsymbol{\zeta})^t\, \pi(\boldsymbol{\zeta}) < \kappa(\boldsymbol{\eta}) - \kappa(\boldsymbol{\zeta})\,,$$

and, for symmetry reasons,

$$(\boldsymbol{\zeta} - \boldsymbol{\eta})^t \, \pi(\boldsymbol{\eta}) \; < \; \kappa(\boldsymbol{\zeta}) - \kappa(\boldsymbol{\eta})$$

(see, for instance, [19, pp. 69/70]). Summation of both inequalities leads to

$$(\boldsymbol{\zeta} - \boldsymbol{\eta})^t \, (\pi(\boldsymbol{\eta}) - \pi(\boldsymbol{\zeta})) < 0 \, .$$

This yields $\pi(\boldsymbol{\zeta}) \neq \pi(\boldsymbol{\eta})$, and π is shown to be one-to-one. By definition, π is onto and thus bijective. The remaining part follows by assertion (b) and the inverse function theorem (see, e.g., [52, p. 221]). □

Examples: $\mathfrak{b}(n_0, \bullet)$, $\mathcal{IN}(\bullet, \bullet)$, $\mathcal{N}(\bullet, \bullet)$

Example 2.57 For $\mathcal{P} = \mathfrak{b}(n_0, \bullet)$, we obtain from Example 2.38 that

$$\kappa(\zeta) = n_0 \ln\left(1 + e^{\zeta}\right) , \qquad \zeta \in \mathbb{R} \, .$$

Hence, the mean value function is

$$\pi : \quad \mathbb{R} \to (0, n_0) : \quad \zeta \mapsto \frac{n_0 \exp\{\zeta\}}{1 + \exp\{\zeta\}}$$

with inverse function

$$\pi^{-1} : \quad (0, n_0) \to \mathbb{R} : \quad t \mapsto \ln\left(\frac{t}{n_0 - t}\right) .$$

Example 2.58 For $\mathcal{P} = \mathcal{IN}(\bullet, \bullet)$, we conclude from Example 2.41 that

$$\kappa(\boldsymbol{\zeta}) = -\frac{\ln(-2\zeta_2)}{2} - 2\sqrt{\zeta_1 \zeta_2} \, , \qquad \boldsymbol{\zeta} = (\zeta_1, \zeta_2)^t \in (-\infty, 0)^2 \, .$$

Hence, the mean value function is

$$\pi : \quad (-\infty, 0)^2 \to \pi((-\infty, 0)^2) : \quad \boldsymbol{\zeta} \mapsto \left(\sqrt{\frac{\zeta_2}{\zeta_1}} , -\frac{1}{2\zeta_2} + \sqrt{\frac{\zeta_1}{\zeta_2}}\right)^t$$

with inverse function

$$\pi^{-1} : \quad \pi((-\infty, 0)^2) \to (-\infty, 0)^2 : \quad \boldsymbol{t} \mapsto \left(\frac{1}{2t_1(1 - t_1 t_2)} , \frac{t_1}{2(1 - t_1 t_2)}\right)^t .$$

Example 2.59 For $\mathcal{P} = \mathcal{N}(\bullet, \bullet)$, we obtain from Example 2.52 that the mean value function is given by

$$\pi: \quad \mathbb{R} \times (-\infty, 0) \to \pi(\mathbb{R} \times (-\infty, 0)): \quad \boldsymbol{\zeta} \mapsto \left(-\frac{\zeta_1}{2\zeta_2}, \frac{\zeta_1^2 - 2\zeta_2}{4\zeta_2^2}\right)^t$$

with inverse function

$$\pi^{-1}: \quad \pi(\mathbb{R} \times (-\infty, 0)) \to \mathbb{R} \times (-\infty, 0): \quad \boldsymbol{t} \mapsto \left(\frac{t_1}{t_2 - t_1^2}, \frac{1}{2(t_1^2 - t_2)}\right)^t.$$

Moreover, we have

$$\pi(\mathbb{R} \times (-\infty, 0)) = \{(x, y)^t \in \mathbb{R}^2 : x^2 < y\}.$$

In Theorem 2.56, the image of the mapping π can be stated explicitly provided that the EF is steep (see [4, p. 117] and [20, p. 71] for the definition and an illustration). The concept of steepness is originally introduced in a more general context for convex functions. Here, for simplicity, we give a definition directly for the full EF with minimal canonical representation.

Definition 2.60 Let $\mathcal{P}$ be a full EF with minimal canonical representation (2.6). $\mathcal{P}$ is called *steep* if, for all $\boldsymbol{\eta} \in \Xi^* \setminus int(\Xi^*)$ and $\boldsymbol{\zeta} \in int(\Xi^*)$, we have

$$\lim_{\alpha \nearrow 1} \frac{\partial}{\partial \alpha} \kappa(\boldsymbol{\zeta}^{(\alpha)}) = \lim_{\alpha \nearrow 1} (\boldsymbol{\eta} - \boldsymbol{\zeta})^t \, \nabla \kappa(\boldsymbol{\zeta}^{(\alpha)}) = \infty, \tag{2.12}$$

where $\boldsymbol{\zeta}^{(\alpha)} = \boldsymbol{\zeta} + \alpha(\boldsymbol{\eta} - \boldsymbol{\zeta})$, $\alpha \in (0, 1)$.

Roughly speaking, Eq. (2.12) ensures that the cumulant function of the EF has infinite slope when moving towards boundary points in Ξ^* on straight lines. A regular EF trivially meets the condition, since such boundary points do not exist in that case.

Lemma 2.61 *Let $\mathcal{P}$ be an EF with minimal canonical representation (2.6). Then, the following implications are true:*

$$\mathcal{P} \text{ is regular} \quad \Rightarrow \quad \mathcal{P} \text{ is steep} \quad \Rightarrow \quad \mathcal{P} \text{ is full} .$$

As pointed out in Example 2.41, the full EF of inverse normal distributions is not regular, but it can be shown to be steep (see [4, p. 117] or [20, p. 72]). An example for a full EF which is not steep is presented in [20, p. 86].

Remark 2.62 In Theorem 2.56, we have

$$\pi(int(\Xi^*)) \subset int(M) , \tag{2.13}$$

where M denotes the convex support of ν^T, i.e., the closed convex hull of the support of ν^T (see, e.g., [37, p. 668]). If $\mathcal{P}$ is steep, then equality holds true in formula (2.13); for a proof, see, e.g., [20, pp. 74/75]. Recall that the support of ν^T coincides with the support of $(P_{\zeta}^*)^T$ for every $\zeta \in \Xi^*$, since these measures are all equivalent; this finding may ease to derive M.

The properties of the mean value function π in Theorem 2.56 allow for the following parametrization of a regular EF.

Definition 2.63 Let $\mathcal{P}$ be a regular EF with minimal canonical representation (2.6). Then,

$$\tilde{P}_m = P^*_{\pi^{-1}(m)} , \qquad m \in \pi(\Xi^*) = int(M)$$

is called the *mean value parametrization* of $\mathcal{P}$, where M is as defined in Remark 2.62.

Some examples illustrate the mean value parametrization of an EF.

Examples: $\mathfrak{poi}(\bullet)$, $\mathcal{N}_k(\bullet, \Sigma_0)$

Example 2.64 According to Example 2.37, $\mathcal{P} = \mathfrak{poi}(\bullet)$ is regular with canonical representation given by the counting densities

$$f_{\zeta}^*(x) = C^*(\zeta)\, e^{\zeta x}\, \frac{1}{x!} , \qquad x \in \mathbb{N}_0 ,$$

with $C^*(\zeta) = \exp\{-e^\zeta\}$ for $\zeta \in \Xi^* = \mathbb{R}$. Hence, the cumulant function is

$$\kappa(\zeta) = e^\zeta\,, \qquad \zeta \in \mathbb{R}\,,$$

and we conclude by Corollary 2.50 that the mean and variance of the statistic $T(x) = x$, $x \in \mathbb{N}_0$, under P^*_ζ are given by

$$E_\zeta[T] = \kappa'(\zeta) = e^\zeta\,,$$

$$\mathrm{Var}_\zeta(T) = \kappa''(\zeta) = e^\zeta\,.$$

Here, the mean value function π is

$$\pi : \mathbb{R} \to (0, \infty) : \zeta \mapsto e^\zeta$$

with inverse function

$$\pi^{-1} : (0, \infty) \to \mathbb{R} : t \mapsto \ln(t)\,.$$

To obtain the mean value parametrization, we set $\zeta = \pi^{-1}(m) = \ln(m)$ in f^*_ζ and arrive at the counting densities

$$\tilde{f}_m(x) = e^{-m}\, m^x \frac{1}{x!}\,, \qquad x \in \mathbb{N}_0\,,$$

for $m \in (0, \infty)$, which is the common representation of $\mathfrak{poi}(\bullet)$ as introduced in Example 2.3. In this parametrization, mean and variance of T under $\tilde{P}_m$ are both equal to m.

Example 2.65 For $\mathcal{P} = \mathcal{N}_k(\bullet, \boldsymbol{\Sigma}_0)$, we obtain from Example 2.54 that the mean value function π and its inverse function π^{-1} are given by

$$\pi : \mathbb{R}^k \to \mathbb{R}^k : \boldsymbol{\mu} \mapsto \boldsymbol{\Sigma}_0^{-1}\boldsymbol{\mu}$$

$$\text{and} \qquad \pi^{-1} : \mathbb{R}^k \to \mathbb{R}^k : \boldsymbol{t} \mapsto \boldsymbol{\Sigma}_0 \boldsymbol{t}\,.$$

To find the mean value parametrization, we set $\boldsymbol{\mu} = \pi^{-1}(\boldsymbol{m}) = \boldsymbol{\Sigma}_0\boldsymbol{m}$ in $f_{\boldsymbol{\mu},\boldsymbol{\Sigma}_0}$ (see Example 2.18) and obtain the Lebesgue densities

$$\tilde{f}_{\boldsymbol{m}}(\boldsymbol{x}) = \exp\left\{-||\boldsymbol{m}||^2_{\boldsymbol{\Sigma}_0^{-1}}/2\right\} e^{\boldsymbol{m}^t\boldsymbol{x}}\, h(\boldsymbol{x})\,, \qquad \boldsymbol{x} \in \mathbb{R}^k\,,$$

for $\boldsymbol{m} \in \mathbb{R}^k$. In this parametrization, mean vector and covariance matrix of $\boldsymbol{T}$ under $\tilde{P}_{\boldsymbol{m}}$ are given by $\boldsymbol{m}$ and $\boldsymbol{\Sigma}_0^{-1}$, respectively. Note that the parametrizations coincide if $\boldsymbol{\Sigma}_0 = \mathbf{E}_k$, i.e., if $\boldsymbol{\Sigma}_0$ is the k-dimensional unit matrix.

Related to the mean value parametrization is the so-called variance function, which leads to a wide range of publications with structural considerations of EFs.

Remark 2.66 An EF $\mathcal{P} = \{P_{\boldsymbol{\zeta}}^* : \boldsymbol{\zeta} \in int(\Xi^*)\}$ with minimal canonical representation (2.6) and $\boldsymbol{T}(\boldsymbol{x}) = \boldsymbol{x}$, $\boldsymbol{x} \in \mathcal{X}$, i.e., with ν-densities

$$\frac{dP_{\boldsymbol{\zeta}}^*}{d\nu}(\boldsymbol{x}) = C^*(\boldsymbol{\zeta})\, e^{\boldsymbol{\zeta}^t \boldsymbol{x}} = e^{\boldsymbol{\zeta}^t \boldsymbol{x} - \kappa(\boldsymbol{\zeta})}\,, \qquad \boldsymbol{x} \in \mathbb{R}^k\,, \tag{2.14}$$

for $\boldsymbol{\zeta} \in int(\Xi^*)$, forms a natural EF with generating measure ν as introduced in [37, Chapter 54] and Remark 2.36. Here, minimality of representation (2.14) ensures that $int(\Xi^*) \neq \emptyset$ and that the support of ν is not contained in an affine hyperplane of $\mathbb{R}^k$. If $\mathcal{P}$ is moreover steep, the *variance function* of $\mathcal{P}$ is defined by

$$V_{\mathcal{P}}(\boldsymbol{m}) = \mathbf{Cov}_{\tilde{P}_{\boldsymbol{m}}}(\boldsymbol{X})\,, \qquad \boldsymbol{m} \in int(M)\,,$$

i.e., $V_{\mathcal{P}}$ maps the mean $\boldsymbol{m}$ of the random vector $\boldsymbol{X}$ to the covariance matrix of $\boldsymbol{X}$ under $\tilde{P}_{\boldsymbol{m}}$, where $int(M)$ is the domain of the means as defined in Remark 2.62 (see, e.g., [37, pp. 669/670]). By Theorem 2.56, we have the identity

$$V_{\mathcal{P}}(\boldsymbol{m}) = \mathbf{H}_{\kappa}(\pi^{-1}(\boldsymbol{m}))\,, \qquad \boldsymbol{m} \in int(M)\,.$$

In Example 2.64, $\mathcal{P}$ forms a natural EF with linear variance function $V_{\mathcal{P}}(m) = m$, $m \in (0, \infty)$. For $\boldsymbol{\Sigma}_0 = \mathbf{E}_k$, the EF $\mathcal{P}$ in Example 2.65 is natural and has constant variance function $V_{\mathcal{P}}(\boldsymbol{m}) = \mathbf{E}_k$, $\boldsymbol{m} \in \mathbb{R}^k$. One motivation for considering variance functions is that it enables to characterize, classify, and construct natural EFs. The interested reader is referred to, e.g., [41], [37, pp. 669/670 and pp. 678–691], and the references therein. A recent overview on the topic is provided in [3].

Chapter 3
Distributional and Statistical Properties

In the third chapter, some further distributional and structural properties of an EF are examined, and basic results for statistical inference in EFs are provided.

3.1 Generating Functions

At the beginning of Sect. 2.2, we have mentioned that the vector $\boldsymbol{T} = (T_1, \ldots, T_k)^t$ of statistics is fundamental in statistical inference. Theorem 2.49 already shows how to derive the moments of $\boldsymbol{T}$ in the EF with natural parametrization. To find the distribution of $\boldsymbol{T}$ under $P^*_{\boldsymbol{\zeta}}$ and for several other applications, it is useful to have simple representations of the *moment generating function* $m_{\boldsymbol{T}}(\boldsymbol{a}) = E_{\boldsymbol{\zeta}}[\exp\{\boldsymbol{a}^t\boldsymbol{T}\}]$, $\boldsymbol{a} \in \mathbb{R}^k$, and the *characteristic function* $\varphi_{\boldsymbol{T}}(\boldsymbol{a}) = E_{\boldsymbol{\zeta}}[\exp\{i\boldsymbol{a}^t\boldsymbol{T}\}]$, $\boldsymbol{a} \in \mathbb{R}^k$, available. These are stated in the following lemma.

Lemma 3.1 *Let $\mathcal{P}$ be an EF with canonical representation (2.6), and let $\boldsymbol{\zeta} \in \Xi$.*

(a) If $A \subset \mathbb{R}^k$ is such that $\boldsymbol{\zeta} + A = \{\boldsymbol{\zeta} + \boldsymbol{a} : \boldsymbol{a} \in A\} \subset \Xi$, then

$$m_{\boldsymbol{T}}(\boldsymbol{a}) = \frac{C^*(\boldsymbol{\zeta})}{C^*(\boldsymbol{\zeta} + \boldsymbol{a})}, \qquad \boldsymbol{a} \in A,$$

where integration has been carried out with respect to $P^*_{\boldsymbol{\zeta}}$.

(b) If the function C^* is extended to the complex set $\{\boldsymbol{\zeta} + i\boldsymbol{a} \in \mathbb{C}^k : \boldsymbol{a} \in \mathbb{R}^k\}$ in a canonical way, then

$$\varphi_{\boldsymbol{T}}(\boldsymbol{a}) = \frac{C^*(\boldsymbol{\zeta})}{C^*(\boldsymbol{\zeta} + i\boldsymbol{a})}, \qquad \boldsymbol{a} \in \mathbb{R}^k,$$

where integration has been carried out with respect to $P^*_{\boldsymbol{\zeta}}$.

S. Bedbur, U. Kamps, *Multivariate Exponential Families: A Concise Guide to Statistical Inference*, SpringerBriefs in Statistics,
https://doi.org/10.1007/978-3-030-81900-2_3

Proof

(a) Let $\boldsymbol{\zeta} \in \Xi$ and $\boldsymbol{\zeta} + A \subset \Xi$. Obviously, we have for $\boldsymbol{a} \in A$

$$\begin{aligned} m_{\boldsymbol{T}}(\boldsymbol{a}) &= E_{\boldsymbol{\zeta}}[e^{\boldsymbol{a}^t \boldsymbol{T}}] = \int e^{\boldsymbol{a}^t \boldsymbol{T}(x)} f_{\boldsymbol{\zeta}}^*(x)\, d\mu(x) \\ &= \frac{C^*(\boldsymbol{\zeta})}{C^*(\boldsymbol{\zeta}+\boldsymbol{a})} \int C^*(\boldsymbol{\zeta}+\boldsymbol{a})\, e^{(\boldsymbol{\zeta}+\boldsymbol{a})^t \boldsymbol{T}(x)}\, h(x)\, d\mu(x) \\ &= \frac{C^*(\boldsymbol{\zeta})}{C^*(\boldsymbol{\zeta}+\boldsymbol{a})} . \end{aligned}$$

(b) The representation is obtained by proceeding as in the proof of statement (a).

□

Examples: $\mathfrak{poi}(\bullet)$, $\mathfrak{b}(n_0, \bullet)$, $\mathfrak{m}(n_0, \bullet)$, $\mathcal{N}(\bullet, \bullet)$, $\mathcal{G}(\bullet, \bullet)$, $\mathcal{N}_k(\bullet, \boldsymbol{\Sigma}_0)$

Example 3.2 For $\mathcal{P} = \mathfrak{poi}(\bullet)$, we have by Example 2.37 that $C^*(\zeta) = \exp\{-e^{\zeta}\}$, $\zeta \in \mathbb{R}$, and $T(x) = x$, $x \in \mathcal{X} = \mathbb{N}_0$. Application of Lemma 3.1(a) then yields

$$m_T(b) = \exp\left\{e^{\zeta}(e^b - 1)\right\}, \qquad b \in \mathbb{R},$$

where integration is with respect to P_{ζ}^*. The transformation $\zeta = \ln(a)$ then gives the moment generating function of T in the original parametrization (see Example 2.3), i.e.,

$$m_T(b) = \exp\left\{a(e^b - 1)\right\}, \qquad b \in \mathbb{R},$$

where integration is with respect to $P_a = \mathfrak{poi}(a)$.

Example 3.3 For $\mathcal{P} = \mathfrak{b}(n_0, \bullet)$, we have by Example 2.38 that $C^*(\zeta) = (1 + \exp\{\zeta\})^{-n_0}$, $\zeta \in \mathbb{R}$, and $T(x) = x$, $x \in \mathcal{X} = \{0, 1, \ldots, n_0\}$. Application of Lemma 3.1(a) then yields

$$m_T(a) = \left(\frac{1 + \exp\{\zeta + a\}}{1 + \exp\{\zeta\}}\right)^{n_0}, \qquad a \in \mathbb{R},$$

where integration is with respect to P_{ζ}^*. The transformation $\zeta = \ln(p/(1-p))$ then gives the moment generating function of T in the original parametrization (see Example 2.4), i.e.,

$$m_T(a) = \left(1 - p + pe^a\right)^{n_0}, \qquad a \in \mathbb{R},$$

where integration is with respect to $P_p = \mathfrak{b}(n_0, p)$.

Example 3.4 For $\mathcal{P} = \mathfrak{m}(n_0, \bullet)$ with minimal canonical representation $\tilde{f}^*_{\boldsymbol{\zeta}}$, $\boldsymbol{\zeta} \in \mathbb{R}^{k-1}$, as shown in Example 2.46, we have $C^*(\boldsymbol{\zeta}) = (1 + \sum_{j=1}^{k-1} \exp\{\zeta_j\})^{-n_0}$ for $\boldsymbol{\zeta} \in \mathbb{R}^{k-1}$ and $\boldsymbol{T}(\boldsymbol{x}) = (x_1, \ldots, x_{k-1})^t$ for $\boldsymbol{x} \in \mathcal{X} = \{(y_1, \ldots, y_k)^t \in \mathbb{N}_0^k : \sum_{i=1}^k y_i = n_0\}$. Application of Lemma 3.1(a) then yields

$$m_{\boldsymbol{T}}(\boldsymbol{a}) = \left(\frac{1 + \sum_{j=1}^{k-1} \exp\{\zeta_j + a_j\}}{1 + \sum_{j=1}^{k-1} \exp\{\zeta_j\}}\right)^{n_0}, \qquad \boldsymbol{a} = (a_1, \ldots, a_{k-1})^t \in \mathbb{R}^{k-1},$$

where integration is with respect to $\tilde{P}^*_{\boldsymbol{\zeta}}$ with counting density $\tilde{f}^*_{\boldsymbol{\zeta}}$. For $k = 2$, we are in the case of Example 3.3.

Example 3.5 In Example 2.39, the canonical representation of $\mathcal{P} = \mathcal{N}(\bullet, \bullet)$ yields

$$C^*(\boldsymbol{\zeta}) = \sqrt{-2\zeta_2} \exp\left\{\frac{\zeta_1^2}{4\zeta_2}\right\}, \qquad \boldsymbol{\zeta} = (\zeta_1, \zeta_2)^t \in \mathbb{R} \times (-\infty, 0),$$

and $\boldsymbol{T}(x) = (T_1(x), T_2(x))^t = (x, x^2)^t$, $x \in \mathbb{R}$. Then, by Lemma 3.1(b), the characteristic function of T_1 is

$$\begin{aligned}
\varphi_{T_1}(a_1) &= \varphi_{\boldsymbol{T}}((a_1, 0)^t) = \frac{C^*(\boldsymbol{\zeta})}{C^*(\boldsymbol{\zeta} + i(a_1, 0)^t)} \\
&= \exp\left\{\frac{\zeta_1^2}{4\zeta_2} - \frac{(\zeta_1 + ia_1)^2}{4\zeta_2}\right\} = \exp\left\{-\frac{i\zeta_1 a_1}{2\zeta_2} + \frac{a_1^2}{4\zeta_2}\right\}, \qquad a_1 \in \mathbb{R},
\end{aligned}$$

where integration is with respect to $P^*_{\boldsymbol{\zeta}}$. In terms of the common parametrization of the univariate normal distribution (see Example 2.10), we find for the characteristic function of a random variable $X = T_1(X) \sim \mathcal{N}(\mu, \sigma^2)$ with $(\zeta_1, \zeta_2) = (\mu/\sigma^2, -1/(2\sigma^2))$ the well known expression

$$\varphi_{T_1}(t) = \exp\left\{i\mu t - \frac{\sigma^2 t^2}{2}\right\}, \qquad t \in \mathbb{R},$$

where integration is with respect to $P_{\mu,\sigma^2} = \mathcal{N}(\mu, \sigma^2)$.

Example 3.6 For $\mathcal{P} = \mathcal{G}(\bullet, \bullet)$, we have by Example 2.40 that $C^*(\boldsymbol{\zeta}) = (-\zeta_1)^{\zeta_2}/\Gamma(\zeta_2)$, $\boldsymbol{\zeta} = (\zeta_1, \zeta_2)^t \in (-\infty, 0) \times (0, \infty)$, and $\boldsymbol{T}(x) = (x, \ln(x))^t$, $x \in (0, \infty)$. Application of Lemma 3.1(a) then yields

$$m_{\boldsymbol{T}}(\boldsymbol{a}) = \frac{\Gamma(\zeta_2 + a_2)}{\Gamma(\zeta_2)} \frac{(-\zeta_1)^{\zeta_2}}{(-\zeta_1 - a_1)^{\zeta_2 + a_2}}$$

for $\boldsymbol{a} = (a_1, a_2)^t \in (-\infty, -\zeta_1) \times (-\zeta_2, \infty)$, where integration is with respect to $P^*_{\boldsymbol{\zeta}}$. The transformation $\zeta_1 = -1/\alpha$, $\zeta_2 = \beta$ then gives the moment generating function of $\boldsymbol{T}$ in the original parametrization (see Example 2.12), i.e.,

$$m_{\boldsymbol{T}}(\boldsymbol{a}) = \frac{\Gamma(\beta + a_2)}{\Gamma(\beta)} \frac{\alpha^{a_2}}{(1 - \alpha a_1)^{\beta + a_2}}, \qquad \boldsymbol{a} \in (-\infty, 1/\alpha) \times (-\beta, \infty),$$

where integration is with respect to $P_{\alpha,\beta} = \mathcal{G}(\alpha, \beta)$.

Example 3.7 For the EF $\mathcal{P} = \mathcal{N}_k(\bullet, \boldsymbol{\Sigma}_0)$ of multivariate normal distributions as in Example 2.18, we have

$$C(\boldsymbol{\mu}) = \exp\left\{-\frac{||\boldsymbol{\mu}||^2_{\boldsymbol{\Sigma}_0}}{2}\right\} = \exp\left\{-\frac{1}{2}\boldsymbol{\mu}^t\boldsymbol{\Sigma}_0^{-1}\boldsymbol{\mu}\right\}, \qquad \boldsymbol{\mu} \in \mathbb{R}^k,$$

and $\boldsymbol{T}(\boldsymbol{x}) = \boldsymbol{\Sigma}_0^{-1}\boldsymbol{x}$, $\boldsymbol{x} \in \mathbb{R}^k$. Hence, by Lemma 3.1(b) with $\boldsymbol{\zeta} = \boldsymbol{\mu}$ and $C^* = C$ (cf. Example 2.54), the characteristic function of $\boldsymbol{T}$ is given by

$$\begin{aligned} \varphi_{\boldsymbol{T}}(\boldsymbol{a}) &= \exp\left\{-\frac{1}{2}\boldsymbol{\mu}^t\boldsymbol{\Sigma}_0^{-1}\boldsymbol{\mu} + \frac{1}{2}(\boldsymbol{\mu} + i\boldsymbol{a})^t\boldsymbol{\Sigma}_0^{-1}(\boldsymbol{\mu} + i\boldsymbol{a})\right\} \\ &= \exp\left\{i\boldsymbol{\mu}^t\boldsymbol{\Sigma}_0^{-1}\boldsymbol{a} - \frac{1}{2}\boldsymbol{a}^t\boldsymbol{\Sigma}_0^{-1}\boldsymbol{a}\right\}, \qquad \boldsymbol{a} \in \mathbb{R}^k, \end{aligned}$$

where integration is with respect to $P_{\boldsymbol{\mu},\boldsymbol{\Sigma}_0} = \mathcal{N}_k(\boldsymbol{\mu}, \boldsymbol{\Sigma}_0)$. This yields the well known expression for the characteristic function of a random vector $\boldsymbol{X} = \boldsymbol{\Sigma}_0\boldsymbol{T}(\boldsymbol{X}) \sim \mathcal{N}_k(\boldsymbol{\mu}, \boldsymbol{\Sigma}_0)$ as

$$\varphi_{\boldsymbol{\Sigma}_0\boldsymbol{T}}(\boldsymbol{t}) = \varphi_{\boldsymbol{T}}(\boldsymbol{\Sigma}_0\boldsymbol{t}) = \exp\left\{i\boldsymbol{\mu}^t\boldsymbol{t} - \frac{1}{2}\boldsymbol{t}^t\boldsymbol{\Sigma}_0\boldsymbol{t}\right\}, \qquad \boldsymbol{t} \in \mathbb{R}^k.$$

It is known in general that if the moment generating function $m_{\boldsymbol{T}}$ of a random vector $\boldsymbol{T}$ with values in $\mathbb{R}^k$ is finite in a neighborhood of $\mathbf{0} \in \mathbb{R}^k$, then all partial derivatives of $m_{\boldsymbol{T}}$ exist finitely, and moments of $\boldsymbol{T}$ can be obtained by calculating respective partial derivatives at $\mathbf{0}$. The logarithm of a moment generating function is called a *cumulant generating function*, and its partial derivatives at $\mathbf{0}$ are termed *cumulants* of $\boldsymbol{T}$, which are applied, for instance, in Edgeworth expansions (see, e.g., [36] and [35]). For further details on moments and cumulants as well as their interrelation, we refer to the literature.

Remark 3.8 In the situation of Lemma 3.1(a) with $k = 1$ (one-parameter case), let $K_T = \ln(m_T)$ denote the cumulant generating function of T. Then, we find the relation

$$K_T(a) = \ln\left(\frac{C^*(\zeta)}{C^*(\zeta + a)}\right) = \kappa(\zeta + a) - \kappa(\zeta), \qquad a \in A,$$

to the cumulant function $\kappa = -\ln(C^*)$ of the EF (see Definition 2.43). If $0 \in int(A)$, the n-th cumulant $\mathcal{K}_T^{(n)}$ of T is defined as the n-th derivative of K_T at 0, i.e., we have

$$\mathcal{K}_T^{(n)} = \frac{\partial^n}{\partial a^n} K_T(a)|_{a=0} = \frac{\partial^n}{\partial \zeta^n}\kappa(\zeta).$$

In particular, we obtain the first two cumulants $\mathcal{K}_T^{(1)}$ and $\mathcal{K}_T^{(2)}$ of T, which are known to give the mean and variance of T under P_ζ^*, as respective derivatives of κ (as already shown in Corollary 2.50).

3.2 Marginal and Conditional Distributions

It is natural to ask whether the EF structure is preserved by considering marginal and conditional distributions. To begin with, the restriction of the sample space to a subset $\mathcal{Y} \subset \mathcal{X}$ yields an EF, again (see, e.g., [44, p. 37]).

Lemma 3.9 *Let $\mathcal{P}$ be an EF with representation (2.1) and $\nu = h\mu$ as in Lemma 2.15. Moreover, let $\mathcal{Y} \in \mathcal{B}$ with $\nu(\mathcal{Y}) > 0$, and let $Q_\vartheta(\cdot) = P_\vartheta(\cdot|\mathcal{Y})$ for $\vartheta \in \Theta$. Then, the family $\{Q_\vartheta : \vartheta \in \Theta\}$ of conditional distributions forms an EF with μ-density*

$$\frac{dQ_\vartheta}{d\mu}(y) = C_{\mathcal{Y}}(\vartheta)\exp\left\{\sum_{j=1}^{k} Z_j(\vartheta)T_j(y)\right\} h(y), \qquad y \in \mathcal{Y},$$

and normalizing constant $C_{\mathcal{Y}}(\vartheta)$ for $\vartheta \in \Theta$.

Proof Let $\vartheta \in \Theta$. Since $\nu(\mathcal{Y}) > 0$, we have $P_\vartheta(\mathcal{Y}) > 0$ by Remark 2.16. Then, for $A \in \mathcal{B} \cap \mathcal{Y}$, we find

$$Q_\vartheta(A) = \frac{P_\vartheta(A \cap \mathcal{Y})}{P_\vartheta(\mathcal{Y})} = \frac{\int_A f_\vartheta \, d\mu}{\int_\mathcal{Y} f_\vartheta \, d\mu},$$

and thus

$$\frac{dQ_\vartheta}{d\mu} = \frac{f_\vartheta}{\int_\mathcal{Y} f_\vartheta \, d\mu},$$

where $\int_\mathcal{Y} f_\vartheta d\mu = C(\vartheta)/C_\mathcal{Y}(\vartheta)$, say. □

Example: $\mathcal{E}(\bullet)$

Example 3.10 Let $\mathcal{P} = \mathcal{E}(\bullet)$, $P_\alpha = \mathcal{E}(\alpha)$ for $\alpha \in (0, \infty)$, and $\mathcal{Y} = [b, \infty)$ for some fixed constant $b \in (0, \infty)$. Then, for $\alpha \in (0, \infty)$, $P_\alpha(\cdot|\mathcal{Y})$ has Lebesgue density

$$C_\mathcal{Y}(\alpha) \exp\left\{-\frac{y}{\alpha}\right\}, \qquad y \in [b, \infty),$$

where

$$C_\mathcal{Y}(\alpha) = \left(\int_b^\infty \exp\left\{-\frac{y}{\alpha}\right\} dy\right)^{-1} = \frac{\exp\{b/\alpha\}}{\alpha}, \qquad \alpha \in (0, \infty).$$

Hence, $\{P_\alpha(\cdot|\mathcal{Y}) : \alpha \in (0, \infty)\}$ is the EF of exponential distributions with location parameter b.

The conditional EF in Lemma 3.9 is not to be mixed up with the truncated EF, which does not form an EF in the proper sense (see Sect. 2.1).

For the EF $\mathcal{P}^T$ of distributions of $\boldsymbol{T}$, the following results for marginal and conditional distributions can be shown; for the proof, see, e.g., [35, pp. 255–257].

Theorem 3.11 *Let $\mathcal{P}$ be an EF with canonical representation (2.6) and $k \geq 2$. Moreover, let $\boldsymbol{U} = (T_1, \ldots, T_r)^t$ and $\boldsymbol{V} = (T_{r+1}, \ldots, T_k)^t$ for some fixed $r \in \{1, \ldots, k-1\}$.*

(a) Let $\zeta_1, \ldots, \zeta_r$ be fixed. Then, there exists a σ-finite measure $Q_{\zeta_1,\ldots,\zeta_r}$ on $\mathbb{B}^{k-r}$ depending on $\zeta_1, \ldots, \zeta_r$, such that the distributions of $\boldsymbol{V}$ form an EF with

densities

$$\frac{d(P_{\boldsymbol{\zeta}}^{*})^{\boldsymbol{V}}}{dQ_{\zeta_1,\ldots,\zeta_r}}(t_{r+1},\ldots,t_k) = C(\boldsymbol{\zeta}) \exp\left\{\sum_{j=r+1}^{k} \zeta_j t_j\right\}, \qquad t_{r+1},\ldots,t_k \in \mathbb{R}. \tag{3.1}$$

(*b*) *There exists a σ-finite measure $\tilde{Q}_{\boldsymbol{v}}$ on $\mathbb{B}^r$, such that the conditional distributions of $\boldsymbol{U}$ given $\boldsymbol{V} = \boldsymbol{v}$ form an EF with densities*

$$\frac{d(P_{\boldsymbol{\zeta}}^{*})^{\boldsymbol{U}|\boldsymbol{V}=\boldsymbol{v}}}{d\tilde{Q}_{\boldsymbol{v}}}(t_1,\ldots,t_r) = C_{\boldsymbol{v}}(\zeta_1,\ldots,\zeta_r) \exp\left\{\sum_{j=1}^{r} \zeta_j t_j\right\}, \qquad t_1,\ldots,t_r \in \mathbb{R},$$

where $C_{\boldsymbol{v}}(\zeta_1,\ldots,\zeta_r)$ denotes a normalizing constant. $\tilde{Q}_{\boldsymbol{v}}$ and $C_{\boldsymbol{v}}(\zeta_1,\ldots,\zeta_r)$ are independent of $\zeta_{r+1},\ldots,\zeta_k$.

We shall highlight the findings in Theorem 3.11 from an inferential perspective. Suppose that we are only interested in estimating the parameters ζ_j, $j \in J$, for some index set $J \subsetneq \{1,\ldots,k\}$. If the parameters ζ_j, $j \notin J$, are assumed to be known, inference may be carried out in the marginal model based on the distribution of $(T_j)_{j\in J}$ forming an EF by varying ζ_j, $j \in J$. However, if ζ_j, $j \notin J$, are unknown, the dominating measure and normalizing constant in the marginal density will be unknown as well, such that inference based on the marginal model will not be feasible or at least gets more involved. In contrast, conditioning $(T_j)_{j\in J}$ on $(T_j)_{j\notin J}$ will eliminate the unknown nuisance parameters ζ_j, $j \notin J$, while maintaining the EF structure of the model.

Remark 3.12 If the density in formula (3.1) does not depend on $\zeta_1,\ldots,\zeta_r$, $\boldsymbol{V}$ is called a *cut* for $\mathcal{P}$ (see, e.g., [37, pp. 673–676], and the references cited therein). Necessary and sufficient conditions for a statistic to be a cut for a (natural) EF can be found in [4, Chapter 10]. For cuts and the related topic of *mixed parametrizations*, the reader is also referred to [44, pp. 240–245] and [20, pp. 78–81].

3.3 Product Measures

We are aiming for statistical inference with EFs in later sections, where we assume to have a sample of independent random variables. Hence, we shall now focus on the corresponding family of product measures. From the respective product densities it becomes clear that the EF structure is preserved for the product case. In what follows, let $\bigotimes_{i=1}^{n} \mathcal{B}_i$ denote the product σ-algebra of the σ-algebras $\mathcal{B}_1,\ldots,\mathcal{B}_n$ and $\bigotimes_{i=1}^{n} Q_i$ denote the product measure of the σ-finite measures $Q_1,\ldots,Q_n$ for $n \in \mathbb{N}$. Moreover, for $n \in \mathbb{N}$, we use the notation $\mathcal{B}^n = \bigotimes_{i=1}^{n} \mathcal{B}$ and $Q^{(n)} = \bigotimes_{i=1}^{n} Q$ for the n-fold product σ-algebra of a σ-algebra $\mathcal{B}$ and the n-fold product measure of a σ-finite measure Q, respectively.

Theorem 3.13

(a) *For $1 \le i \le n$, let $(\mathcal{X}_i, \mathcal{B}_i)$ be a measurable space and $\mathcal{P}_i = \{P_{\vartheta_i;i} : \vartheta_i \in \Theta_i\}$ be an EF of distributions on $\mathcal{B}_i$ dominated by a σ-finite measure μ_i. Then, the class*

$$\left\{ \bigotimes_{i=1}^{n} P_{\vartheta_i;i} \, : \, \vartheta_i \in \Theta_i \, , 1 \le i \le n \right\}$$

of product measures on $\bigotimes_{i=1}^{n} \mathcal{B}_i$ forms an EF dominated by $\bigotimes_{i=1}^{n} \mu_i$.

(b) *Let $\mathcal{P}$ be an EF with representation (2.1). For $n \in \mathbb{N}$, let $P_{\vartheta}^{(n)} = \bigotimes_{i=1}^{n} P_{\vartheta}$ for $P_{\vartheta} \in \mathcal{P}$. Then, the class*

$$\mathcal{P}^{(n)} = \left\{ P_{\vartheta}^{(n)} : \vartheta \in \Theta \right\}$$

of product measures on $\mathcal{B}^n$ forms an EF dominated by $\mu^{(n)}$, where, for $\vartheta \in \Theta$, a $\mu^{(n)}$-density of $P_{\vartheta}^{(n)}$ is given by

$$f_{\vartheta}^{(n)}(\tilde{\boldsymbol{x}}) = C(\vartheta)^n \exp\left\{ \sum_{j=1}^{k} Z_j(\vartheta) T_j^{(n)}(\tilde{\boldsymbol{x}}) \right\} \left(\prod_{i=1}^{n} h(x^{(i)}) \right)$$

with statistics

$$T_j^{(n)}(\tilde{\boldsymbol{x}}) = \sum_{i=1}^{n} T_j(x^{(i)}) \, , \qquad 1 \le j \le k \, , \tag{3.2}$$

for $\tilde{\boldsymbol{x}} = (x^{(1)}, \ldots, x^{(n)}) \in \mathcal{X}^n$.

Consequently, the joint distribution of independent random variables $X_1, \ldots, X_n$ forms an EF if the distribution of X_i, $1 \le i \le n$, forms an EF. In Theorem 3.13, case (a) corresponds to a sample of independent not necessarily identically distributed (inid) random variables; case (b) then refers to the situation of an independent and identically distributed (iid) sample.

Examples: $\mathsf{poi}(\bullet)$, $\mathcal{N}(\bullet, \bullet)$, $\mathcal{N}_k(\bullet, \boldsymbol{\Sigma}_0)$

Example 3.14 Let $X_1, \ldots, X_n$ be independent random variables with $X_i \sim \mathsf{poi}(a_i)$ for $1 \le i \le n$ as in Example 2.3. Then, the distribution of $\tilde{\boldsymbol{X}} = (X_1, \ldots, X_n)$ forms a multiparameter EF with representation (2.1) given by $\mu = \mu_{\mathbb{N}_0}^{(n)}$, $k = n$,

$$C(\boldsymbol{a}) = \exp\left\{ -\sum_{i=1}^{n} a_i \right\} , \qquad Z_j(\boldsymbol{a}) = \ln(a_j) \, , \quad 1 \le j \le n \, ,$$

for $\boldsymbol{a} = (a_1, \ldots, a_n)^t \in (0, \infty)^n$, and

$$T_j(\tilde{\boldsymbol{x}}) = x_j, \quad 1 \le j \le n, \qquad h(\tilde{\boldsymbol{x}}) = \prod_{i=1}^{n} \frac{1}{x_i!}$$

for $\tilde{\boldsymbol{x}} = (x_1, \ldots, x_n) \in \mathbb{N}_0^n$. Clearly, this EF has order n and is regular. On the other hand, by assuming that $a_1 = \cdots = a_n$, we are in the iid situation with an EF of order 1. Obviously, we can generate EFs with one parameter up to n parameters, here. Now, suppose that the parameters $a_1, \ldots, a_n$ are connected via a log-linear link function, i.e., we set $\ln(a_j) = \zeta_1 + \zeta_2 v_j$, $1 \le j \le n$, where ζ_1 and ζ_2 are real-valued parameters and $v_1, \ldots, v_n$ are fixed real numbers, which are not all identical. By inserting, the distribution of $\tilde{\boldsymbol{X}}$ turns out to form a regular EF of order 2 with canonical representation (2.6), where

$$C^*(\boldsymbol{\zeta}) = \exp\left\{-\sum_{i=1}^{n} e^{\zeta_1 + \zeta_2 v_i}\right\}, \qquad \boldsymbol{\zeta} = (\zeta_1, \zeta_2)^t \in \mathbb{R}^2,$$

and $\boldsymbol{T}(\tilde{\boldsymbol{x}}) = (\sum_{i=1}^n x_i, \sum_{i=1}^n v_i x_i)^t$ for $\tilde{\boldsymbol{x}} = (x_1, \ldots, x_n) \in \mathbb{N}_0^n$ (see [44, p. 35]).

Example 3.15 Let $X_1, \ldots, X_{n_1}$ be an iid sample from $\mathcal{N}(\mu_1, \sigma_1^2)$ and $Y_1, \ldots, Y_{n_2}$ be an iid sample from $\mathcal{N}(\mu_2, \sigma_2^2)$ as introduced in Example 2.10. Moreover, let the samples be independent. Then, the distribution of $(X_1, \ldots, X_{n_1}, Y_1, \ldots, Y_{n_2})$ forms an EF with representation (2.1) given by $\mu = \lambda_{\mathbb{R}}^{n_1+n_2}$, $k = 4$,

$$C(\boldsymbol{\vartheta}) = \left(\sigma_1^2\right)^{-n_1/2} \left(\sigma_2^2\right)^{-n_2/2} \exp\left\{-\frac{n_1\mu_1^2}{2\sigma_1^2} - \frac{n_2\mu_2^2}{2\sigma_2^2}\right\},$$

$$\boldsymbol{Z}(\boldsymbol{\vartheta}) = \left(\frac{\mu_1}{\sigma_1^2}, \frac{\mu_2}{\sigma_2^2}, -\frac{1}{2\sigma_1^2}, -\frac{1}{2\sigma_2^2}\right)^t,$$

for $\boldsymbol{\vartheta} = (\mu_1, \mu_2, \sigma_1^2, \sigma_2^2)^t \in \mathbb{R}^2 \times (0, \infty)^2$, and

$$\boldsymbol{T}(\tilde{\boldsymbol{x}}) = \left(\sum_{i=1}^{n_1} x_i, \sum_{j=1}^{n_2} y_j, \sum_{i=1}^{n_1} x_i^2, \sum_{j=1}^{n_2} y_j^2\right)^t, \qquad h(\tilde{\boldsymbol{x}}) = \left(\frac{1}{\sqrt{2\pi}}\right)^{n_1+n_2},$$

for $\tilde{\boldsymbol{x}} = (x_1, \ldots, x_{n_1}, y_1, \ldots, y_{n_2}) \in \mathbb{R}^{n_1+n_2}$. Clearly, the EF has order 4 and is regular. Now, suppose that $\sigma_1^2 = \sigma_2^2 = \sigma^2$, say, i.e., we have a common-scale model. By inserting, the distribution of $\tilde{\boldsymbol{X}}$ turns out to form an EF with mappings

$$C(\tilde{\boldsymbol{\vartheta}}) = \left(\sigma^2\right)^{-(n_1+n_2)/2} \exp\left\{-\frac{n_1\mu_1^2 + n_2\mu_2^2}{2\sigma^2}\right\},$$

$$\boldsymbol{Z}(\tilde{\boldsymbol{\vartheta}}) = \left(\frac{\mu_1}{\sigma^2}, \frac{\mu_2}{\sigma^2}, -\frac{1}{2\sigma^2}\right)^t,$$

for $\tilde{\boldsymbol{\vartheta}} = (\mu_1, \mu_2, \sigma^2)^t \in \mathbb{R}^2 \times (0, \infty)$, and

$$\boldsymbol{T}(\tilde{\boldsymbol{x}}) = \left(\sum_{i=1}^{n_1} x_i, \sum_{j=1}^{n_2} y_j, \sum_{i=1}^{n_1} x_i^2 + \sum_{j=1}^{n_2} y_j^2\right)^t,$$

for $\tilde{\boldsymbol{x}} = (x_1, \ldots, x_{n_1}, y_1, \ldots, y_{n_2}) \in \mathbb{R}^{n_1+n_2}$. This is a regular EF of order 3. In contrast, the common-location assumption $\mu_1 = \mu_2$ leads to a curved EF of order 4 (see also [35, pp. 87/88]).

Example 3.16 Let $X_1, \ldots, X_n$ be independent random variables with $X_i \sim \mathcal{N}(\mu_i, \sigma_0^2)$, $i \in \{1, \ldots, n\}$, for some fixed variance $\sigma_0^2 > 0$. Then, by Theorem 3.13(a), the joint distributions of $X_1, \ldots, X_n$ form an EF of distributions on $(\mathbb{R}^n, \mathbb{B}^n)$ with parameters $\mu_1, \ldots, \mu_n \in \mathbb{R}$.

Now, let $\boldsymbol{X}^{(1)}, \ldots, \boldsymbol{X}^{(m)}$ be iid random vectors following a multivariate normal distribution with mean vector $\boldsymbol{\mu} = (\mu_1, \ldots, \mu_n)^t \in \mathbb{R}^n$ and fixed positive definite covariance matrix $\boldsymbol{\Sigma}_0 \in \mathbb{R}^{n\times n}$, i.e., $\boldsymbol{X}^{(i)} \sim \mathcal{N}_n(\boldsymbol{\mu}, \boldsymbol{\Sigma}_0)$, $i \in \{1, \ldots, m\}$. Then, by Theorem 3.13(b), the joint distributions of $\boldsymbol{X}^{(1)}, \ldots, \boldsymbol{X}^{(m)}$ form an EF of distributions on $(\mathbb{R}^{mn}, \mathbb{B}^{mn})$ with parameters $\mu_1, \ldots, \mu_n \in \mathbb{R}$.

Based on Theorem 3.13, the latter examples show the flexibility of constructing EFs. Suppose that, in the situation of Example 3.16, we want to have a 3-parameter EF of distributions on $(\mathbb{R}^6, \mathbb{B}^6)$. This is achieved, for instance, by choosing $n = 6$ in the independent case while assuming $\mu_2 = \mu_3$ and $\mu_4 = \mu_5 = \mu_6$, or by setting $n = 3$ and $m = 2$ in the iid case.

Given the iid situation, several properties of the EF are transferred to the product EF. In what follows, let $\boldsymbol{T}^{(n)} = (T_1^{(n)}, \ldots, T_k^{(n)})^t$ with $T_j^{(n)}$, $1 \leq j \leq k$, as defined in formula (3.2), be the vector of statistics for the n-fold product case, $n \in \mathbb{N}$.

Corollary 3.17 *Let $\mathcal{P}$ be an EF with representation (2.1), and let $\mathcal{P}^{(n)}$, $n \in \mathbb{N}$, denote the corresponding EF of n-fold product measures. Then, $ord(\mathcal{P}^{(n)}) = ord(\mathcal{P})$. Moreover, if $\mathcal{P}$ is full (regular, steep), so is $\mathcal{P}^{(n)}$.*

Proof Considering $\boldsymbol{T}^{(n)}$ as function of iid random variables $X_1, \ldots, X_n \sim P_\vartheta$, it follows that

$$\mathbf{Cov}_{P_\vartheta^{(n)}}(\boldsymbol{T}^{(n)}) = n\,\mathbf{Cov}_{P_\vartheta}(\boldsymbol{T}) .$$

Hence, $\mathcal{P}$ and $\mathcal{P}^{(n)}$ have the same order by applying Lemma 2.26 and Theorem 2.23. Moreover, by Fubini's theorem, we have for $\boldsymbol{\zeta} \in \mathbb{R}^k$ that

$$\int e^{\boldsymbol{\zeta}^t \boldsymbol{T}^{(n)}} h_n \, d\mu^{(n)} = \left(\int e^{\boldsymbol{\zeta}^t \boldsymbol{T}} h \, d\mu \right)^n ,$$

where $h_n(\tilde{\boldsymbol{x}}) = \prod_{i=1}^n h(x^{(i)})$ for $\tilde{\boldsymbol{x}} = (x^{(1)}, \ldots, x^{(n)}) \in \mathcal{X}^n$, such that the natural parameter spaces of $\mathcal{P}^{(n)}$ and $\mathcal{P}$ coincide. Trivially, $\mathcal{P}^{(n)}$ is then full (regular) if $\mathcal{P}$ is full (regular). Finally, since the cumulant function of $\mathcal{P}^{(n)}$ is given by $n\kappa$, $\mathcal{P}^{(n)}$ is steep if $\mathcal{P}$ is steep. □

Note that Lemma 2.17 and Theorem 3.13(b) with $\boldsymbol{T}(x) = x$, $x \in \mathcal{X}$, imply that the distribution of a sum of iid random variables forms an EF if this is the case for the distribution of the summands (for more details, see [37, pp. 670–673]). In other words, the EF structure is preserved for the family of n-fold convolutions. Here, the cumulant function for the n-fold convolution family is given by $n\kappa$, $n \in \mathbb{N}$. For the steep natural EF $\mathcal{P}$ with ν-densities (2.14), this finding suggests the construction of a more general family of distributions. Let $\Lambda \subset (0, \infty)$ denote the set of all parameters λ, for which $\lambda\kappa$ is the cumulant function of a natural EF generated by some measure ν_λ on $\mathbb{B}^k$. Then,

$$\mathcal{D} = \{P^*_{\boldsymbol{\zeta},\lambda} : \boldsymbol{\zeta} \in int(\Xi^*),\ \lambda \in \Lambda\}$$

is called the *exponential dispersion model* associated with $\mathcal{P}$, where a ν_λ-density of $P^*_{\boldsymbol{\zeta},\lambda}$ is given by

$$\frac{dP^*_{\boldsymbol{\zeta},\lambda}}{d\nu_\lambda}(\boldsymbol{x}) = e^{\boldsymbol{\zeta}^t \boldsymbol{x} - \lambda\kappa(\boldsymbol{\zeta})} , \qquad \boldsymbol{x} \in \mathbb{R}^k ,$$

for $\boldsymbol{\zeta} \in int(\Xi^*)$ and $\lambda \in \Lambda$. $\mathcal{D}$ is the union of the natural EFs $\{P^*_{\boldsymbol{\zeta},\lambda} : \boldsymbol{\zeta} \in int(\Xi^*)\}$ with variance functions $V_\lambda(\boldsymbol{m}) = \lambda V_{\mathcal{P}}(\boldsymbol{m}/\lambda)$, $\boldsymbol{m} \in int(\lambda M)$, for $\lambda \in \Lambda$ (see Remark 2.66). The parameter $1/\lambda$ is called the *dispersion parameter*, and Λ is also referred to as the Jørgensen set in the literature. For an extensive account on the model, see [29]. Applications of exponential dispersion models can be found, for instance, in [3] and the references cited therein. For their particular use in generalized linear models and actuarial risk theory, see, e.g., [61, 23, 56, 30].

3.4 Sufficiency and Completeness

The concepts of sufficiency and completeness of a statistic for a family of distributions is fundamental in various aspects of statistical inference as, for example, the derivation of optimal point estimators and statistical tests. Roughly speaking, a sufficient statistic contains and summarizes all information in the data about the underlying true distribution, and it comprises no redundant information if it is complete, too. In general, sufficiency is introduced via conditional expectations and probabilities (see, e.g., [40, pp. 36–44]). Here, for short, we introduce sufficiency by means of the form of the density functions in the family, which is known as the Neyman criterion (see, e.g., [40, pp. 44–46]).

Definition 3.18 Let $(\mathcal{X}, \mathcal{B})$ be a measurable space and $\mathcal{P} = \{P_\vartheta : \vartheta \in \Theta\}$ be a family of distributions on $\mathcal{B}$ dominated by a σ-finite measure μ. Moreover, let $\boldsymbol{T} : (\mathcal{X}, \mathcal{B}) \to (\mathcal{Y}, \mathcal{C})$ be a statistic.

(a) $\boldsymbol{T}$ is called *sufficient for* $\vartheta \in \Theta$ if there exist a function $h : (\mathcal{X}, \mathcal{B}) \to (\mathbb{R}^1, \mathbb{B}^1)$ and functions $q_\vartheta : (\mathcal{Y}, \mathcal{C}) \to (\mathbb{R}^1, \mathbb{B}^1)$, $\vartheta \in \Theta$, such that a μ-density of P_ϑ is of the form

$$\frac{dP_\vartheta}{d\mu}(x) = q_\vartheta(\boldsymbol{T}(x))\, h(x)\,, \qquad x \in \mathcal{X}\,, \tag{3.3}$$

for all $\vartheta \in \Theta$.

(b) $\boldsymbol{T}$ is called *minimal sufficient for* $\vartheta \in \Theta$ if $\boldsymbol{T}$ is sufficient for $\vartheta \in \Theta$ and factorizes over any other sufficient statistic, i.e., for every statistic $\tilde{\boldsymbol{T}} : (\mathcal{X}, \mathcal{B}) \to (\tilde{\mathcal{Y}}, \tilde{\mathcal{C}})$ being sufficient for $\vartheta \in \Theta$, there exist a function $q : (\tilde{\mathcal{Y}}, \tilde{\mathcal{C}}) \to (\mathcal{Y}, \mathcal{C})$ and a set $N \in \mathcal{B}$ with $P_\vartheta(N) = 0$ for all $\vartheta \in \Theta$, such that

$$\boldsymbol{T} = q \circ \tilde{\boldsymbol{T}} \qquad \text{on } N^c.$$

A sufficient statistic allows for reduction of the data without a loss of information meaning that $\boldsymbol{T}(x)$ contains all information in x about ϑ. The main issue in formula (3.3) is that the term $q_\vartheta(\boldsymbol{T}(x))$ depends on the observation x only through $\boldsymbol{T}(x)$. A minimal sufficient statistic is as simple as possible in the sense of Definition 3.18(b).

Definition 3.19 Let $(\mathcal{X}, \mathcal{B})$ be a measurable space and $\mathcal{P} = \{P_\vartheta : \vartheta \in \Theta\}$ be a family of distributions on $\mathcal{B}$.

(a) $\mathcal{P}$ is called *(boundedly) complete* if, for every (bounded) function $r : (\mathcal{X}, \mathcal{B}) \to (\mathbb{R}^1, \mathbb{B}^1)$, the following implication holds:

$$\int r \, dP_\vartheta = 0 \quad \text{for all } \vartheta \in \Theta$$

$$\Rightarrow \quad \text{there exists a set } N \in \mathcal{B} \text{ with } P_\vartheta(N) = 0 \text{ for all } \vartheta \in \Theta$$

$$\text{and } r(x) = 0 \text{ for all } x \in N^c .$$

(b) A statistic $\boldsymbol{T} : (\mathcal{X}, \mathcal{B}) \to (\mathcal{Y}, \mathcal{C})$ is called *(boundedly) complete for* $\vartheta \in \Theta$ if $\mathcal{P}^{\boldsymbol{T}} = \{P_\vartheta^{\boldsymbol{T}} : \vartheta \in \Theta\}$ is (boundedly) complete.

The completeness of a statistic refers to the richness of the underlying family $\mathcal{P}$ of distributions. By definition, every complete statistic is boundedly complete. In an EF, a (minimal) sufficient and complete statistic is easily found, which means an important advantage in statistical inference.

Theorem 3.20 *Let $\mathcal{P}$ be an EF with representation (2.1). Then, we have the following properties:*

(a) The vector $\boldsymbol{T} = (T_1, \ldots, T_k)^t$ is sufficient for $\vartheta \in \Theta$.
(b) If $Z_1, \ldots, Z_k$ are affinely independent, then $\boldsymbol{T}$ is minimal sufficient for $\vartheta \in \Theta$.
(c) If $int(\boldsymbol{Z}(\Theta)) \neq \emptyset$, then $\boldsymbol{T}$ is complete for $\vartheta \in \Theta$.

Statement (a) in Theorem 3.20 directly follows by setting $q_\vartheta(\boldsymbol{t}) = C(\vartheta) \exp\{\boldsymbol{Z}(\vartheta)^t \boldsymbol{t}\}$, $\boldsymbol{t} \in \mathbb{R}^k$, in Eq. (3.3), and it holds true in any EF without imposing further conditions on $Z_1, \ldots, Z_k$. A proof of statement (b) can be found, for instance, in [39, p. 39] and [50, pp. 25/26]. Statement (c) can be shown by using characteristic functions and the uniqueness theorem (see, e.g., [40, pp. 116/117], [50, pp. 26/27], or [20, p. 43]).

The property of an EF to be full along with a minimal representation (see Definitions 2.35 and 2.20) has direct applications for the statistic $\boldsymbol{T}$, namely, it is minimal sufficient and complete.

Corollary 3.21 *Let $\mathcal{P}$ be a full EF with minimal representation (2.1). Then, $\boldsymbol{T} = (T_1, \ldots, T_k)^t$ is minimal sufficient and complete for ϑ.*

Proof The assertion follows from Theorem 3.20, Lemma 2.42, and Theorem 2.23. □

Note that the dimension of the vector $\boldsymbol{T}^{(n)}$ of statistics related to the product case is the same for all $n \in \mathbb{N}$ (see Theorem 3.13(b)). Hence, in the iid case, sampling from an EF does not increase the dimension of the sufficient statistic.

Examples: $\mathfrak{poi}(\bullet)$, $\mathfrak{b}(n_0, \bullet)$, $\mathfrak{nb}(r_0, \bullet)$, $\mathfrak{m}(n_0, \bullet)$, $\mathcal{E}(\bullet)$, $\mathfrak{g}(\bullet, \bullet)$, $\mathcal{G}(\bullet, \bullet)$, $\mathcal{N}(\bullet, \bullet)$, $\mathcal{N}_k(\bullet, \Sigma_0)$

Example 3.22 Let $\mathcal{P}$ be any of the EFs $\mathfrak{poi}(\bullet)$, $\mathfrak{b}(n_0, \bullet)$, $\mathfrak{nb}(r_0, \bullet)$, or $\mathcal{E}(\bullet)$ introduced in Examples 2.3, 2.4, 2.5, and 2.12. Moreover, let $X_1, \ldots, X_n$ be an iid sample from $P_\vartheta \in \mathcal{P}$. Then, by Theorem 3.20,

$$T^{(n)}(\tilde{\boldsymbol{x}}) = \sum_{i=1}^{n} x_i \,, \qquad \tilde{\boldsymbol{x}} = (x_1, \ldots, x_n) \in \mathcal{X}^n \,,$$

is minimal sufficient and complete for ϑ.

Example 3.23 Let $\mathcal{P}$ be the EF $\mathfrak{g}(\bullet, \bullet)$ or $\mathcal{G}(\bullet, \bullet)$ defined in Examples 2.7 and 2.12. Moreover, let $X_1, \ldots, X_n$ be an iid sample from $P_{\boldsymbol{\vartheta}} \in \mathcal{P}$. Then, by Theorem 3.20,

$$\boldsymbol{T}^{(n)}(\tilde{\boldsymbol{x}}) = \left(\sum_{i=1}^{n} x_i \,, \sum_{i=1}^{n} \ln(x_i) \right)^t \,, \qquad \tilde{\boldsymbol{x}} = (x_1, \ldots, x_n) \in \mathcal{X}^n \,,$$

is minimal sufficient and complete for $\boldsymbol{\vartheta}$.

Example 3.24 Let $\boldsymbol{X}^{(1)}, \ldots, \boldsymbol{X}^{(n)}$ be an iid sample from $\mathfrak{m}(n_0, \boldsymbol{p}) \in \mathfrak{m}(n_0, \bullet)$ as introduced in Example 2.8. Then, by Theorem 3.20 and Example 2.46,

$$\tilde{\boldsymbol{T}}^{(n)}(\tilde{\boldsymbol{x}}) = \sum_{i=1}^{n} (x_1^{(i)}, \ldots, x_{k-1}^{(i)})^t \,, \qquad \tilde{\boldsymbol{x}} = (\boldsymbol{x}^{(1)}, \ldots, \boldsymbol{x}^{(n)}) \in \mathcal{X}^n \,,$$

$$\boldsymbol{x}^{(i)} = (x_1^{(i)}, \ldots, x_k^{(i)})^t \in \mathcal{X} \,, \; 1 \le i \le n \,,$$

is minimal sufficient and complete for $\boldsymbol{p}$.

Example 3.25 Let $X_1, \ldots, X_n$ be an iid sample from $\mathcal{N}(\mu, \sigma^2) \in \mathcal{N}(\bullet, \bullet)$ as introduced in Example 2.10. Then, by Theorem 3.20 and Example 2.27,

$$\boldsymbol{T}^{(n)}(\tilde{\boldsymbol{x}}) = \left(\sum_{i=1}^{n} x_i\,,\, \sum_{i=1}^{n} x_i^2\right)^t, \qquad \tilde{\boldsymbol{x}} = (x_1, \ldots, x_n) \in \mathbb{R}^n,$$

is minimal sufficient and complete for $(\mu, \sigma^2)^t$.

Example 3.26 Let $\boldsymbol{X}^{(1)}, \ldots, \boldsymbol{X}^{(n)}$ be an iid sample from $\mathcal{N}_k(\boldsymbol{\mu}, \boldsymbol{\Sigma}_0) \in \mathcal{N}_k(\bullet, \boldsymbol{\Sigma}_0)$ as introduced in Example 2.18. Then, by Theorem 3.20 and Example 2.28,

$$\boldsymbol{T}^{(n)}(\tilde{\boldsymbol{x}}) = \sum_{i=1}^{n} \boldsymbol{x}^{(i)}, \qquad \tilde{\boldsymbol{x}} = (\boldsymbol{x}^{(1)}, \ldots, \boldsymbol{x}^{(n)}) \in (\mathbb{R}^k)^n,$$

is minimal sufficient and complete for $\boldsymbol{\mu}$.

Remark 3.27 For the curved EF introduced in Definition 2.32, statements (a) and (b) of Theorem 3.20 are true. Completeness of $\boldsymbol{T}$, however, may or may not be the case. In [50, pp. 28–31], examples for complete and non-complete curved EFs are shown and sufficient conditions are given for $\boldsymbol{T}$ to be not complete or not even boundedly complete.

3.5 Score Statistic and Information Matrix

The Fisher information matrix is a measure for the amount of information a random variable/vector contains about the true underlying parameter. It appears, for instance, in the context of point estimation and allows for defining efficient and asymptotically efficient estimators.

Definition 3.28 Let $(\mathcal{X}, \mathcal{B})$ be a measurable space and $\mathcal{P} = \{P_\vartheta = f_\vartheta \mu : \vartheta \in \Theta\}$, $\Theta \subset \mathbb{R}^k$ open, be a family of distributions on $\mathcal{B}$ dominated by a σ-finite measure μ. If all appearing derivatives (with respect to ϑ) and integrals

(continued)

Definition 3.28 (continued)
(with respect to P_ϑ) exist, then

$$\mathbf{I}(\vartheta) = E_{P_\vartheta}[\boldsymbol{U}_\vartheta \boldsymbol{U}_\vartheta^t] \qquad \text{with} \quad \boldsymbol{U}_\vartheta = \nabla \ln(f_\vartheta)$$

is called the *Fisher information matrix* of $\mathcal{P}$ at $\vartheta \in \Theta$. The random vector $\boldsymbol{U}_\vartheta$ is referred to as the *score statistic* at $\vartheta \in \Theta$.

In an EF with natural parametrization, differentiability of the densities with respect to $\boldsymbol{\zeta}$ is guaranteed by Corollary 2.50, and the score statistic and Fisher information matrix are readily obtained.

Theorem 3.29 *Let $\mathcal{P}$ be an EF with canonical representation (2.6), and let $\boldsymbol{\zeta} \in int(\Xi)$. Then,*

$$\boldsymbol{U}_\zeta = \boldsymbol{T} - E_\zeta[\boldsymbol{T}],$$

$$\mathbf{I}(\boldsymbol{\zeta}) = \mathbf{Cov}_\zeta(\boldsymbol{T}).$$

In particular, all entries in $\mathbf{I}(\boldsymbol{\zeta})$ are finite, i.e., $[\mathbf{I}(\boldsymbol{\zeta})]_{i,j} < \infty$, $1 \le i, j \le k$. If $ord(\mathcal{P}) = k$, then $\mathbf{I}(\boldsymbol{\zeta}) > 0$.

Proof Let $\boldsymbol{\zeta} \in int(\Xi)$. By Corollary 2.50,

$$\boldsymbol{U}_\zeta = \nabla \ln(\exp\{\boldsymbol{\zeta}^t \boldsymbol{T} - \kappa(\boldsymbol{\zeta})\} h) = \boldsymbol{T} - E_\zeta[\boldsymbol{T}].$$

Hence, $\mathbf{I}(\boldsymbol{\zeta}) = \mathbf{Cov}_\zeta(\boldsymbol{T})$. Moreover, from Theorem 2.49, all entries in $\mathbf{I}(\boldsymbol{\zeta})$ are finite. If $ord(\mathcal{P}) = k$, then $\mathbf{I}(\boldsymbol{\zeta}) > 0$ by Theorem 2.23 and Lemma 2.26. □

Moreover, the following simple formula for the Fisher information matrix results from Corollary 2.50.

Corollary 3.30 *Let $\mathcal{P}$ be an EF with canonical representation (2.6). Then,*

$$\mathbf{I}(\boldsymbol{\zeta}) = \mathbf{H}_\kappa(\boldsymbol{\zeta}), \quad \boldsymbol{\zeta} \in int(\Xi).$$

For one-parameter EFs with canonical representation and $\zeta \in int(\Xi)$, the Fisher information is simply given by the second derivative of κ at ζ.

Examples: $\mathfrak{poi}(\bullet)$, $\mathfrak{nb}(r_0, \bullet)$, $\mathcal{N}(\bullet, \bullet)$, $\mathcal{G}(\bullet, \bullet)$, $\mathcal{N}_k(\bullet, \boldsymbol{\Sigma}_0)$

Example 3.31 For $\mathcal{P} = \mathfrak{poi}(\bullet)$, Corollary 3.30 and Example 2.64 directly yield $I(\zeta) = e^{\zeta}$ for $\zeta \in \mathbb{R}$.

Example 3.32 For $\mathcal{P} = \mathfrak{nb}(r_0, \bullet)$, Corollary 3.30 and Example 2.51 directly yield

$$I(\zeta) = \frac{r_0 \exp\{\zeta\}}{(1 - \exp\{\zeta\})^2}, \qquad \zeta \in (-\infty, 0).$$

Example 3.33 For $\mathcal{P} = \mathcal{N}(\bullet, \bullet)$, Corollary 3.30 and Example 2.52 yield

$$\mathbf{I}(\boldsymbol{\zeta}) = \begin{pmatrix} -\frac{1}{2\zeta_2} & \frac{\zeta_1}{2\zeta_2^2} \\ \frac{\zeta_1}{2\zeta_2^2} & \frac{1}{2\zeta_2^2} - \frac{\zeta_1^2}{2\zeta_2^3} \end{pmatrix} = \frac{1}{2\zeta_2^3} \begin{pmatrix} -\zeta_2^2 & \zeta_1\zeta_2 \\ \zeta_1\zeta_2 & \zeta_2 - \zeta_1^2 \end{pmatrix}$$

for $\boldsymbol{\zeta} = (\zeta_1, \zeta_2)^t \in \mathbb{R} \times (-\infty, 0)$.

Example 3.34 For $\mathcal{P} = \mathcal{G}(\bullet, \bullet)$, Corollary 3.30 and Example 2.53 directly yield

$$\mathbf{I}(\boldsymbol{\zeta}) = \begin{pmatrix} \frac{\zeta_2}{\zeta_1^2} & -\frac{1}{\zeta_1} \\ -\frac{1}{\zeta_1} & \psi_1(\zeta_2) \end{pmatrix}, \qquad \boldsymbol{\zeta} = (\zeta_1, \zeta_2)^t \in (-\infty, 0) \times (0, \infty),$$

where $\psi_1 = \psi'$ denotes the trigamma function.

Example 3.35 For $\mathcal{P} = \mathcal{N}_k(\bullet, \boldsymbol{\Sigma}_0)$, Corollary 3.30 and Example 2.54 directly yield

$$\mathbf{I}(\boldsymbol{\mu}) = \boldsymbol{\Sigma}_0^{-1}, \qquad \boldsymbol{\mu} \in \mathbb{R}^k.$$

The Fisher information matrix generally depends on the parametrization of the distribution family. In the situation of Definition 3.28, let $\mathbf{I}(\boldsymbol{\vartheta})$ exist for $\boldsymbol{\vartheta} \in \Theta$. Moreover, let $\Delta \subset \mathbb{R}^q$, $q \leq k$, be open, and let $\Psi : \Delta \to \Theta$ be a one-to-one and continuously differentiable function with Jacobian matrix $\mathbf{D}_{\Psi}(\boldsymbol{\eta}) \in \mathbb{R}^{k \times q}$ of full rank for all $\boldsymbol{\eta} \in \Delta$. Then, the score statistic and Fisher information matrix at $\boldsymbol{\eta} \in \Delta$

of the family $\{\tilde{P}_\eta : \eta \in \Delta\} \subset \mathcal{P}$ with parametrization $\tilde{P}_\eta = P_{\Psi(\eta)}$, $\eta \in \Delta$, are given by

$$\begin{aligned}\tilde{\mathbf{U}}_\eta &= \mathbf{D}_\Psi(\eta)^t\, \mathbf{U}_{\Psi(\eta)}\,,\\ \tilde{\mathbf{I}}(\eta) &= \mathbf{D}_\Psi(\eta)^t\, \mathbf{I}(\Psi(\eta))\, \mathbf{D}_\Psi(\eta)\,. \end{aligned} \tag{3.4}$$

Example

Example 3.36 Let $\mathcal{P}$ be a regular EF with minimal canonical representation (2.6), and let $\pi : \Xi^* \to \pi(\Xi^*)$ be the mean value function as defined in Theorem 2.56 with Jacobian matrix $\mathbf{D}_\pi(\boldsymbol{\zeta}) = \mathbf{Cov}_{\boldsymbol{\zeta}}(\boldsymbol{T})$ for $\boldsymbol{\zeta} \in \Xi^*$. Then, by using Theorem 3.29, formula (3.4) with $\Psi = \pi^{-1}$, and $\mathbf{D}_{\pi^{-1}}(\boldsymbol{m}) = [\mathbf{D}_\pi(\pi^{-1}(\boldsymbol{m}))]^{-1}$, the Fisher information matrix of $\mathcal{P}$ corresponding to the mean value parametrization $\tilde{P}_{\boldsymbol{m}} = P^*_{\pi^{-1}(\boldsymbol{m})}$, $\boldsymbol{m} \in \pi(\Xi^*)$, is given by

$$\begin{aligned}\tilde{\mathbf{I}}(\boldsymbol{m}) &= \mathbf{D}_{\pi^{-1}}(\boldsymbol{m})^t\, \mathbf{I}(\pi^{-1}(\boldsymbol{m}))\, \mathbf{D}_{\pi^{-1}}(\boldsymbol{m})\\ &= [\mathbf{Cov}_{\pi^{-1}(\boldsymbol{m})}(\boldsymbol{T})]^{-1}\, \mathbf{Cov}_{\pi^{-1}(\boldsymbol{m})}(\boldsymbol{T})\, [\mathbf{Cov}_{\pi^{-1}(\boldsymbol{m})}(\boldsymbol{T})]^{-1}\\ &= [\mathbf{Cov}_{\pi^{-1}(\boldsymbol{m})}(\boldsymbol{T})]^{-1}\\ &= [\mathbf{Cov}_{\tilde{P}_{\boldsymbol{m}}}(\boldsymbol{T})]^{-1}\,, \qquad \boldsymbol{m} \in \pi(\Xi^*)\,.\end{aligned}$$

3.6 Divergence and Distance Measures

Entropy measures as, for instance, the Shannon entropy defined by $H(P) = -E_P[\ln(f)]$ for a distribution P with μ-density f, measure the disorder and uncertainty of distributions. Closely related are *divergence measures*, which quantify the 'distance' of two distributions in some family $\mathcal{P}$ in a certain sense (see, e.g., [57] and [48]). In statistical inference, they serve to construct statistical tests or confidence regions for underlying parameters. If the distributions in $\mathcal{P}$ are dominated by a σ-finite measure μ, various divergence measures have been introduced by means of the corresponding densities. Some important examples are the *Kullback-Leibler divergence*

$$D_{KL}(P_1, P_2) = \int f_1 \ln\left(\frac{f_1}{f_2}\right) d\mu\,,$$

the *Jeffrey distance* $D_J(P_1, P_2) = D_{KL}(P_1, P_2) + D_{KL}(P_2, P_1)$, the *Rényi divergence*

$$D_{R_q}(P_1, P_2) = \frac{1}{q(q-1)} \ln\left(\int f_1^q f_2^{1-q}\, d\mu\right), \qquad q \in \mathbb{R} \setminus \{0, 1\},$$

the *Cressie-Read divergence*

$$D_{CR_q}(P_1, P_2) = \frac{1}{q(q-1)} \int f_1 \left(\left(\frac{f_1}{f_2}\right)^{q-1} - 1\right) d\mu, \qquad q \in \mathbb{R} \setminus \{0, 1\},$$

and the *Hellinger metric*

$$D_H(P_1, P_2) = \left(\int \left(\sqrt{f_1} - \sqrt{f_2}\right)^2 d\mu\right)^{1/2}$$

for $P_i = f_i\mu \in \mathcal{P}$, $i = 1, 2$, provided that the respective expressions are defined and the integrals finitely exist. If $\mathcal{P} = \{P_\vartheta : \vartheta \in \Theta\}$ is a parametric family of distributions, it is convenient to use the parameters as arguments and briefly write, e.g., $D_{KL}(\vartheta_1, \vartheta_2)$ for $D_{KL}(P_{\vartheta_1}, P_{\vartheta_2})$, $\vartheta_1, \vartheta_2 \in \Theta$; note that then $D_{KL}(\vartheta_1, \vartheta_2) = 0$ implies $\vartheta_1 = \vartheta_2$ if the parameter $\vartheta \in \Theta$ is identifiable (see Lemma 2.30).

The EF structure admits simple formulas for various divergence measures as indicated in Lemma 3.37 and Corollary 3.39. Note that the Kullback-Leibler divergence, which can be considered as an expected log-likelihood ratio, is a starting point for many statistical procedures. Under common assumptions, we obtain a simple representation in EFs (see [20, pp. 174–178]). This representation is used in [33] in a two-class classification procedure within an EF, where classes are defined by means of left-sided Kullback-Leibler balls.

Lemma 3.37 *Let $\mathcal{P}$ be a full EF with minimal canonical representation (2.6). Then, for $\boldsymbol{\zeta}, \boldsymbol{\eta} \in int(\Xi^*)$, we have*

$$D_{KL}(\boldsymbol{\zeta}, \boldsymbol{\eta}) = \kappa(\boldsymbol{\eta}) - \kappa(\boldsymbol{\zeta}) + (\boldsymbol{\zeta} - \boldsymbol{\eta})^t \pi(\boldsymbol{\zeta}),$$

$$D_J(\boldsymbol{\zeta}, \boldsymbol{\eta}) = (\boldsymbol{\zeta} - \boldsymbol{\eta})^t (\pi(\boldsymbol{\zeta}) - \pi(\boldsymbol{\eta})).$$

Proof For $\boldsymbol{\zeta}, \boldsymbol{\eta} \in int(\Xi^*)$, we have by Theorem 2.56

$$\begin{aligned} D_{KL}(\boldsymbol{\zeta}, \boldsymbol{\eta}) &= \int \left(\ln(f_{\boldsymbol{\zeta}}^*) - \ln(f_{\boldsymbol{\eta}}^*)\right) f_{\boldsymbol{\zeta}}^*\, d\mu \\ &= \int \left((\boldsymbol{\zeta} - \boldsymbol{\eta})^t \boldsymbol{T} - \kappa(\boldsymbol{\zeta}) + \kappa(\boldsymbol{\eta})\right) f_{\boldsymbol{\zeta}}^*\, d\mu \end{aligned}$$

$$= \kappa(\boldsymbol{\eta}) - \kappa(\boldsymbol{\zeta}) + (\boldsymbol{\zeta} - \boldsymbol{\eta})^t E_{\boldsymbol{\zeta}}[\boldsymbol{T}]$$

$$= \kappa(\boldsymbol{\eta}) - \kappa(\boldsymbol{\zeta}) + (\boldsymbol{\zeta} - \boldsymbol{\eta})^t \pi(\boldsymbol{\zeta}).$$

From this, the representation of D_J is obvious. □

The Rényi divergence, Cressie-Read divergence, Hellinger metric, and other divergences are functions of the quantity $A_q(P_1, P_2) = \int f_1^q f_2^{1-q}\, d\mu$, which has a nice representation in EFs for $q \in (0, 1)$ (see, e.g., [43, 60]).

Lemma 3.38 *Let $\mathcal{P}$ be a full EF with minimal canonical representation (2.6). Then, for $\boldsymbol{\zeta}, \boldsymbol{\eta} \in \Xi^*$ and $q \in (0, 1)$, we have*

$$A_q(\boldsymbol{\zeta}, \boldsymbol{\eta}) = \exp\{\kappa(q\boldsymbol{\zeta} + (1-q)\boldsymbol{\eta}) - (q\kappa(\boldsymbol{\zeta}) + (1-q)\kappa(\boldsymbol{\eta}))\}.$$

Proof Let $\boldsymbol{\zeta}, \boldsymbol{\eta} \in \Xi^*$ and $q \in (0, 1)$. Then,

$$A_q(\boldsymbol{\zeta}, \boldsymbol{\eta}) = \int (f_{\boldsymbol{\zeta}}^*)^q\, (f_{\boldsymbol{\eta}}^*)^{1-q}\, d\mu$$

$$= \int \exp\left\{(q\boldsymbol{\zeta} + (1-q)\boldsymbol{\eta})^t\, \boldsymbol{T} - (q\kappa(\boldsymbol{\zeta}) + (1-q)\kappa(\boldsymbol{\eta}))\right\} h\, d\mu$$

$$= \exp\{\kappa(q\boldsymbol{\zeta} + (1-q)\boldsymbol{\eta}) - (q\kappa(\boldsymbol{\zeta}) + (1-q)\kappa(\boldsymbol{\eta}))\}.$$

□

Recall that the cumulant function κ is convex (see Theorem 2.44). The logarithm of $A_q(\boldsymbol{\zeta}, \boldsymbol{\eta})$ in Lemma 3.38 is just the difference of κ evaluated at a convex combination of $\boldsymbol{\zeta}$ and $\boldsymbol{\eta}$ and the respective convex combination of $\kappa(\boldsymbol{\zeta})$ and $\kappa(\boldsymbol{\eta})$.

Corollary 3.39 *Let $\mathcal{P}$ be a full EF with minimal canonical representation (2.6). Then, for $\boldsymbol{\zeta}, \boldsymbol{\eta} \in \Xi^*$ and $q \in (0, 1)$, we have*

$$D_{R_q}(\boldsymbol{\zeta}, \boldsymbol{\eta}) = \frac{\kappa(q\boldsymbol{\zeta} + (1-q)\boldsymbol{\eta}) - (q\kappa(\boldsymbol{\zeta}) + (1-q)\kappa(\boldsymbol{\eta}))}{q(q-1)},$$

$$D_{CR_q}(\boldsymbol{\zeta}, \boldsymbol{\eta}) = \frac{\exp\{\kappa(q\boldsymbol{\zeta} + (1-q)\boldsymbol{\eta}) - (q\kappa(\boldsymbol{\zeta}) + (1-q)\kappa(\boldsymbol{\eta}))\} - 1}{q(q-1)},$$

$$D_H(\boldsymbol{\zeta}, \boldsymbol{\eta}) = \left(2 - 2\exp\left\{\kappa\left(\frac{\boldsymbol{\zeta} + \boldsymbol{\eta}}{2}\right) - \frac{\kappa(\boldsymbol{\zeta}) + \kappa(\boldsymbol{\eta})}{2}\right\}\right)^{1/2}.$$

Proof The assertion immediately follows from Lemma 3.38, since $D_{R_q} = (\ln A_q)/[q(q-1)]$, $D_{CR_q} = (A_q - 1)/[q(q-1)]$, and $D_H = (2 - 2A_{1/2})^{1/2}$. □

Remark 3.40 Every divergence measure D, say, of D_{KL}, D_J, D_{R_q}, D_{CR_q}, and D_H in Lemma 3.37 and Corollary 3.39 satisfies the properties that, for any $\boldsymbol{\zeta}, \boldsymbol{\eta} \in int(\Xi^*)$, $D(\boldsymbol{\zeta}, \boldsymbol{\eta}) \geq 0$ and

$$D(\boldsymbol{\zeta}, \boldsymbol{\eta}) = 0 \quad \Leftrightarrow \quad \boldsymbol{\zeta} = \boldsymbol{\eta}\,.$$

Moreover, D_J and D_H are symmetric. Beyond that, D_H meets the triangle inequality and therefore defines a metric on $int(\Xi^*) \times int(\Xi^*)$.

Example: $\mathcal{N}_k(\bullet, \boldsymbol{\Sigma}_0)$

Example 3.41 In the minimal canonical representation of $\mathcal{N}_k(\bullet, \boldsymbol{\Sigma}_0)$ in Example 2.65, the cumulant function and mean value function are given by $\kappa(\boldsymbol{\mu}) = ||\boldsymbol{\mu}||^2_{\boldsymbol{\Sigma}_0}/2$ and $\pi(\boldsymbol{\mu}) = \boldsymbol{\Sigma}_0^{-1}\boldsymbol{\mu}$ for $\boldsymbol{\mu} \in \mathbb{R}^k$. Hence, by Lemma 3.37,

$$\begin{aligned} D_{KL}(\boldsymbol{\mu}, \boldsymbol{\eta}) &= \frac{||\boldsymbol{\mu} - \boldsymbol{\eta}||^2_{\boldsymbol{\Sigma}_0}}{2}\,, \\ D_J(\boldsymbol{\mu}, \boldsymbol{\eta}) &= ||\boldsymbol{\mu} - \boldsymbol{\eta}||^2_{\boldsymbol{\Sigma}_0}\,, \end{aligned}$$

for $\boldsymbol{\mu}, \boldsymbol{\eta} \in \mathbb{R}^k$. Moreover, we have for $q \in (0, 1)$ that

$$\kappa(q\boldsymbol{\mu} + (1-q)\boldsymbol{\eta}) - (q\kappa(\boldsymbol{\mu}) + (1-q)\kappa(\boldsymbol{\eta})) = \frac{q(q-1)||\boldsymbol{\mu} - \boldsymbol{\eta}||^2_{\boldsymbol{\Sigma}_0}}{2}\,,$$

which, by using Corollary 3.39 gives

$$\begin{aligned} D_{R_q}(\boldsymbol{\mu}, \boldsymbol{\eta}) &= \frac{||\boldsymbol{\mu} - \boldsymbol{\eta}||^2_{\boldsymbol{\Sigma}_0}}{2}\,, \\ D_{CR_q}(\boldsymbol{\mu}, \boldsymbol{\eta}) &= \frac{1}{q(q-1)}\left(\exp\left\{\frac{q(q-1)||\boldsymbol{\mu} - \boldsymbol{\eta}||^2_{\boldsymbol{\Sigma}_0}}{2}\right\} - 1\right), \end{aligned}$$

and, by setting $q = 1/2$,

$$D_H(\boldsymbol{\mu}, \boldsymbol{\eta}) = \left(2 - 2\exp\left\{-\frac{||\boldsymbol{\mu} - \boldsymbol{\eta}||^2_{\boldsymbol{\Sigma}_0}}{8}\right\}\right)^{1/2},$$

for $\boldsymbol{\mu}, \boldsymbol{\eta} \in \mathbb{R}^k$. Hence, $D_{KL}(\boldsymbol{\mu}, \boldsymbol{\eta})$, $D_J(\boldsymbol{\mu}, \boldsymbol{\eta})$, $D_{R_q}(\boldsymbol{\mu}, \boldsymbol{\eta})$, $D_{CR_q}(\boldsymbol{\mu}, \boldsymbol{\eta})$, and $D_H(\boldsymbol{\mu}, \boldsymbol{\eta})$ each admit a representation as $h(||\boldsymbol{\mu} - \boldsymbol{\eta}||^2_{\boldsymbol{\Sigma}_0})$ for some increasing function $h : [0, \infty) \to [0, \infty)$.

The above representations of divergences can be applied to develop statistical procedures such as confidence regions (see, e.g., [60]). By using the EF structure, simple formulas for other related quantities may be derived as well. In the full EF with minimal canonical representation (2.6) , the *weighted Matusita affinity*

$$\rho_n(\boldsymbol{\zeta}^{(1)},\ldots,\boldsymbol{\zeta}^{(n)}) = \int \left(\prod_{i=1}^{n} f^*_{\boldsymbol{\zeta}^{(i)}}\right)^{w_i} d\mu\,, \qquad \boldsymbol{\zeta}^{(1)},\ldots,\boldsymbol{\zeta}^{(n)} \in \Xi^*\,,$$

with positive weights $w_1,\ldots,w_n$ satisfying $\sum_{i=1}^n w_i = 1$ and $n \geq 2$ is given by

$$\rho_n(\boldsymbol{\zeta}^{(1)},\ldots,\boldsymbol{\zeta}^{(n)}) = \exp\left\{\kappa\left(\sum_{i=1}^{n} w_i \boldsymbol{\zeta}^{(i)}\right) - \sum_{i=1}^{n} w_i \kappa(\boldsymbol{\zeta}^{(i)})\right\}$$

(cf. Lemma 3.38); it can be applied, e.g., to construct a homogeneity test with null hypothesis $\boldsymbol{\zeta}^{(1)} = \cdots = \boldsymbol{\zeta}^{(n)}$ or to decide in a discriminant problem (see [25, 42, 34]).

Chapter 4
Parameter Estimation

In this chapter, parameter estimation is discussed when the underlying parametric model forms an EF. For this, we focus on the natural parametrization of the EF according to Definition 2.35, i.e., $\mathcal{P} = \{P^*_{\boldsymbol{\zeta}} : \boldsymbol{\zeta} \in \Xi\}$ with μ-densities

$$f^*_{\boldsymbol{\zeta}}(\boldsymbol{x}) = \frac{dP^*_{\boldsymbol{\zeta}}}{d\mu}(\boldsymbol{x}) = C^*(\boldsymbol{\zeta}) \exp\left\{\sum_{j=1}^{k} \zeta_j T_j(\boldsymbol{x})\right\} h(\boldsymbol{x})$$
$$= e^{\boldsymbol{\zeta}^t \boldsymbol{T}(\boldsymbol{x}) - \kappa(\boldsymbol{\zeta})} h(\boldsymbol{x}), \qquad \boldsymbol{x} \in \mathcal{X}, \tag{4.1}$$

for $\boldsymbol{\zeta} \in \Xi$, where $\emptyset \neq \Xi \subset \Xi^*$. To estimate $\boldsymbol{\zeta}$ or, more generally, a parameter $\gamma(\boldsymbol{\zeta})$, $\boldsymbol{\zeta} \in \Xi$, we will assume to have observations $\boldsymbol{x}^{(i)}$ considered realizations of iid random variables $\boldsymbol{X}^{(i)}$ with distribution $P^*_{\boldsymbol{\zeta}} \in \mathcal{P}$ for $i \in I \subset \mathbb{N}$. Every measurable function of $\boldsymbol{X}^{(i)}$, $i \in I$, with values in Ξ is then called an *estimator* of $\boldsymbol{\zeta}$ (in Ξ based on $\boldsymbol{X}^{(i)}$, $i \in I$); an estimator of $\gamma(\boldsymbol{\zeta})$, $\boldsymbol{\zeta} \in \Xi$, or, for short, of γ is a measurable function of $\boldsymbol{X}^{(i)}$, $i \in I$, with values in $\gamma(\Xi)$. Here, all random variables $\boldsymbol{X}^{(i)}$, $i \in I$, are formally defined on the probability space $(\Omega, \mathcal{A}, \mathbb{P}_{\boldsymbol{\zeta}})$, i.e., we have

$$\mathbb{P}^{\boldsymbol{X}^{(i)}}_{\boldsymbol{\zeta}} = P^*_{\boldsymbol{\zeta}}, \qquad i \in I.$$

Moreover, the notation $\mathbb{E}_{\boldsymbol{\zeta}}[\cdot]$, $\mathbb{V}\mathrm{ar}_{\boldsymbol{\zeta}}(\cdot)$, and $\mathbb{C}\mathrm{ov}_{\boldsymbol{\zeta}}(\cdot)$ for the mean, variance, and covariance (matrix) is used when integration is with respect to $\mathbb{P}_{\boldsymbol{\zeta}}$.

S. Bedbur, U. Kamps, *Multivariate Exponential Families: A Concise Guide to Statistical Inference*, SpringerBriefs in Statistics,
https://doi.org/10.1007/978-3-030-81900-2_4

4.1 Maximum Likelihood Estimation

The maximum likelihood method, where, given some observation x of a random variable X with density function $f_{\boldsymbol{\zeta}}^*$, we want to assign a global maximum point of $f_{\boldsymbol{\zeta}}^*(x)$, as a function of $\boldsymbol{\zeta}$, to an estimate of $\boldsymbol{\zeta}$, is closely connected to the study of EFs. Under mild conditions and in the case of Lebesgue density functions, the unique existence of the maximum likelihood estimator can be guaranteed. For counting densities, existence is an issue, while uniqueness is ensured.

Definition 4.1 Let $x \in \mathcal{X}$ be a realization of $X \sim P_{\boldsymbol{\zeta}}^*$. Every parameter in Ξ that maximizes the *likelihood function*

$$L(\boldsymbol{\zeta}; x) = f_{\boldsymbol{\zeta}}^*(x), \quad \boldsymbol{\zeta} \in \Xi,$$

is called a *maximum likelihood estimate* (ML estimate) of $\boldsymbol{\zeta}$ in Ξ based on x.

Equivalently and usually analytically simpler, one may maximize the *log-likelihood function*

$$\ell = \ln(L)$$

to find the ML estimate(s). From formula (4.1), the log-likelihood function in our model is

$$\ell(\boldsymbol{\zeta}; x) = \boldsymbol{\zeta}^t \boldsymbol{T}(x) - \kappa(\boldsymbol{\zeta}) + \ln(h(x)), \qquad \boldsymbol{\zeta} \in \Xi.$$

Hence, the aim is to maximize the expression

$$\boldsymbol{\zeta}^t \boldsymbol{T}(x) - \kappa(\boldsymbol{\zeta})$$

with respect to $\boldsymbol{\zeta}$ in Ξ. For this, it will be convenient to consider the natural extension $\tilde{\kappa}$ of κ with domain $\mathbb{R}^k$ as introduced in Lemma 2.45 and the respective extension $\tilde{\ell}$ of ℓ to $\mathbb{R}^k$ by setting $\tilde{\ell}(\boldsymbol{\zeta}; x) = -\infty$ for $\boldsymbol{\zeta} \in \mathbb{R}^k \setminus \Xi^*$. For a simple notation, these extensions are again denoted by κ and ℓ in the following. Theorem 2.44, Lemma 2.45, and Theorem 2.56 directly yield some useful properties of ℓ.

Lemma 4.2 *Let $\mathcal{P}$ be a full EF with minimal canonical representation (4.1). Then, we have for every $x \in \mathcal{X}$:*

(a) $\ell(\cdot; x)$ *is strictly concave on* Ξ^*.

(b) $\ell(\cdot; x)$ *is upper semi-continuous, i.e.,*

$$\limsup_{\eta \to \zeta} \ell(\eta; x) \leq \ell(\zeta; x) \quad \text{for every } \zeta \in \mathbb{R}^k.$$

(c) $\ell(\cdot; x)$ *is continuously differentiable on* $int(\Xi^*)$ *with derivative*

$$\nabla \ell(\zeta; x) = T(x) - \pi(\zeta), \qquad \zeta \in int(\Xi^*),$$

where π *is the mean value function introduced in Theorem 2.56.*

Note that in Lemma 4.2 the mean value function $\pi : int(\Xi^*) \to \pi(int(\Xi^*))$, defined by $\pi(\zeta) = E_\zeta[T]$ for $\zeta \in int(\Xi^*)$, is bijective with $\pi(int(\Xi^*)) \subset int(M)$, where M denotes the convex support of ν^T (see Theorem 2.56 and Remark 2.62). If $\mathcal{P}$ is moreover steep, we have

$$\pi(int(\Xi^*)) = int(M).$$

Now, we have the following fundamental theorem for steep EFs (see [4, p. 151]).

Theorem 4.3 *Let* $\mathcal{P}$ *be a steep EF with minimal canonical representation (4.1), and let* $x \in \mathcal{X}$ *be a given realization of the random variable X with distribution* $P_\zeta^* \in \mathcal{P}$. *Then, the ML estimate of* ζ *in* Ξ^* *based on x exists if and only if*

$$T(x) \in \pi(int(\Xi^*)) \quad (= int(M)).$$

If it exists, it is uniquely determined and given by $\pi^{-1}(T(x))$.

Proof First, we show that the maximum of $\ell = \ell(\cdot; x)$ cannot be attained at a boundary point of Ξ^*. Let $\eta \in \Xi^* \setminus int(\Xi^*)$, $\zeta \in int(\Xi^*)$, and $\zeta^{(\alpha)} = \zeta + \alpha(\eta - \zeta) \in int(\Xi^*)$, $\alpha \in [0, 1)$. By Lemma 4.2,

$$\begin{aligned} \liminf_{\alpha \nearrow 1} \ell(\zeta^{(\alpha)}) &\geq \liminf_{\alpha \nearrow 1} [\ell(\zeta) + \alpha(\ell(\eta) - \ell(\zeta))] \\ &= \ell(\eta) \geq \limsup_{\alpha \nearrow 1} \ell(\zeta^{(\alpha)}), \end{aligned}$$

i.e., $\lim_{\alpha \nearrow 1} \ell(\zeta^{(\alpha)}) = \ell(\eta)$. Moreover, since $\mathcal{P}$ is steep,

$$\lim_{\alpha \nearrow 1} \frac{\partial}{\partial \alpha} \ell(\zeta^{(\alpha)}) = \lim_{\alpha \nearrow 1} \left[(\eta - \zeta)^t T(x) - \frac{\partial}{\partial \alpha} \kappa(\zeta^{(\alpha)}) \right] = -\infty,$$

such that there exists some $\tilde{\alpha} \in (0, 1)$ with $\ell(\zeta^{(\tilde{\alpha})}) > \ell(\eta)$. Hence, if ℓ has a maximum, it is attained on $int(\Xi^*)$ and necessary a solution of the likelihood equation

$$\mathbf{0} = \nabla \ell(\zeta) = T(x) - \pi(\zeta).$$

In case of $\boldsymbol{T}(x) \in \pi(int(\Xi^*))$, this equation has the only solution $\pi^{-1}(\boldsymbol{T}(x))$, which is then also the unique ML estimate of $\boldsymbol{\zeta}$ in Ξ^* based on x. Otherwise, an ML estimate in Ξ^* based on x does not exist. □

Remark 4.4 In Theorem 4.3, the ML estimate of $\boldsymbol{\zeta}$ in Ξ^* based on a single observation of $X \sim P_{\boldsymbol{\zeta}}^*$ exists with probability

$$P_{\boldsymbol{\zeta}}^*(\boldsymbol{T} \in \pi(int(\Xi^*))) = P_{\boldsymbol{\zeta}}^*(\boldsymbol{T} \in int(M)).$$

Since $\nu^{\boldsymbol{T}}(M^c) = 0$ as well as $\nu^{\boldsymbol{T}}$ and $(P_{\boldsymbol{\zeta}}^*)^{\boldsymbol{T}}$ are equivalent measures by Remark 2.16 and Lemma 2.17, it follows that

$$P_{\boldsymbol{\zeta}}^*(\boldsymbol{T} \notin M) = 0 \qquad \text{for } \boldsymbol{\zeta} \in \Xi^*.$$

Hence, the ML estimate of $\boldsymbol{\zeta}$ in Ξ^* exists with $P_{\boldsymbol{\zeta}}^*$-probability 1 if and only if $\boldsymbol{T}$ lies on the boundary of M with $P_{\boldsymbol{\zeta}}^*$-probability 0. In particular, this is the case if the distribution of $\boldsymbol{T}$ has a Lebesgue density, since the boundary of any convex set in $\mathbb{R}^k$ has Lebesgue measure 0.

Based on an iid sample from $P_{\boldsymbol{\zeta}}^*$, we arrive at the following version of Theorem 4.3.

Corollary 4.5 *Let $\mathcal{P}$ be a steep EF with minimal canonical representation (4.1). Moreover, let $X^{(1)}, \ldots, X^{(n)}$ be an iid sample from the distribution $P_{\boldsymbol{\zeta}}^* \in \mathcal{P}$, and let $x^{(1)}, \ldots, x^{(n)}$ denote realizations of $X^{(1)}, \ldots, X^{(n)}$. Then, the ML estimate of $\boldsymbol{\zeta}$ in Ξ^* based on $x^{(1)}, \ldots, x^{(n)}$ exists if and only if*

$$\frac{1}{n}\sum_{i=1}^{n} \boldsymbol{T}(x^{(i)}) \in \pi(int(\Xi^*)) \qquad (= int(M)). \tag{4.2}$$

If the ML estimate exists, it is uniquely determined and given by

$$\pi^{-1}\left(\frac{1}{n}\sum_{i=1}^{n} \boldsymbol{T}(x^{(i)})\right).$$

Proof By using Theorem 3.13 and Corollary 3.17, we may apply Theorem 4.3 to the EF $\mathcal{P}^{(n)}$ of distributions of $(X^{(1)}, \ldots, X^{(n)})$. By doing so, $\boldsymbol{T}$ and π have to be replaced by $\boldsymbol{T}^{(n)}$ and $n\pi$. The assertion then follows from

$$\boldsymbol{T}^{(n)}(x^{(1)}, \ldots, x^{(n)}) \in (n\pi)(int(\Xi^*)) \qquad \Leftrightarrow \qquad \frac{1}{n}\sum_{i=1}^{n} \boldsymbol{T}(x^{(i)}) \in \pi(int(\Xi^*)).$$

□

Notation 4.6 If, in the situation of Corollary 4.5, condition (4.2) is true with $(P^*_\zeta)^{(n)}$-probability 1, the *maximum likelihood estimator* (MLE) of ζ in Ξ^* based on $X^{(1)}, \dots, X^{(n)}$, which then uniquely exists $\mathbb{P}_\zeta$-a.s., is denoted by

$$\hat{\zeta}^{(n)} = \pi^{-1}\left(\frac{1}{n}\sum_{i=1}^{n} T(X^{(i)})\right). \qquad (4.3)$$

Examples: $\mathfrak{poi}(\bullet)$, $\mathfrak{b}(n_0, \bullet)$, $\mathcal{N}(\bullet, \bullet)$, $\mathcal{N}_k(\bullet, \Sigma_0)$

Example 4.7 From Example 2.64 for $\mathcal{P} = \mathfrak{poi}(\bullet)$, we have $T(x) = x$ for $x \in \mathbb{N}_0$ and $\pi(\zeta) = \exp\{\zeta\}$ for $\zeta \in \Xi^* = \mathbb{R}$. Here, $\pi(int(\Xi^*)) = (0, \infty)$. Now, let $X_1, \dots, X_n$ be an iid sample from P^*_ζ, and let $x_1, \dots, x_n \in \mathbb{N}_0$ denote realizations of $X_1, \dots, X_n$. Then,

$$\frac{1}{n}\sum_{i=1}^{n} x_i \notin (0, \infty) \qquad \Leftrightarrow \qquad x_1 = \cdots = x_n = 0\,.$$

Hence, by Corollary 4.5, an ML estimate of ζ based on $x_1, \dots, x_n \in \mathbb{N}_0$ does not exist if $x_1 = \cdots = x_n = 0$. In any other case,

$$\ln\left(\frac{1}{n}\sum_{i=1}^{n} x_i\right)$$

is the unique ML estimate. The probability for the non-existence of the ML estimate is given by

$$\mathbb{P}_\zeta(X_1 = 0, \dots, X_n = 0) = \exp\left\{-ne^\zeta\right\}, \qquad \zeta \in \mathbb{R},$$

and converges to 0 for $n \to \infty$.

Example 4.8 From Example 2.57 for $\mathcal{P} = \mathfrak{b}(n_0, \bullet)$, we have $T(x) = x$ for $x \in \{0, 1, \dots, n_0\}$, $\Xi^* = \mathbb{R}$, and $\pi(\Xi^*) = (0, n_0)$. Now, let $X_1, \dots, X_n$ be an iid sample from P^*_ζ, and let $x_1, \dots, x_n \in \{0, 1, \dots, n_0\}$ denote realizations of

$X_1, \ldots, X_n$. Then,

$$\frac{1}{n}\sum_{i=1}^{n} x_i \notin (0, n_0) \quad \Leftrightarrow \quad (x_1 = \cdots = x_n = 0 \ \vee \ x_1 = \cdots = x_n = n_0)$$

Hence, by Corollary 4.5, an ML estimate of ζ based on $x_1, \ldots, x_n \in \{0, 1 \ldots, n_0\}$ does not exist if $x_1 = \cdots = x_n = 0$ or $x_1 = \cdots = x_n = n_0$. In any other case,

$$\pi^{-1}\left(\frac{1}{n}\sum_{i=1}^{n} x_i\right) = \ln\left(\frac{\sum_{i=1}^{n} x_i}{n_0 n - \sum_{i=1}^{n} x_i}\right)$$

is the unique ML estimate. The probability for the non-existence of the ML estimate is given by

$$\begin{aligned} &\mathbb{P}_\zeta(\{X_1 = \cdots = X_n = 0\} \cup \{X_1 = \cdots = X_n = n_0\}) \\ &= \left(\frac{1}{1+\exp\{\zeta\}}\right)^{n_0 n} + \left(\frac{\exp\{\zeta\}}{1+\exp\{\zeta\}}\right)^{n_0 n} \end{aligned}$$

and converges to 0 for $n \to \infty$.

Example 4.9 From Example 2.59 for $\mathcal{P} = \mathcal{N}(\bullet, \bullet)$, we have $\boldsymbol{T}(x) = (x, x^2)^t$ for $x \in \mathbb{R}$, $\Xi^* = \mathbb{R} \times (-\infty, 0)$, and

$$\pi(\Xi^*) = \{(x, y)^t \in \mathbb{R}^2 : x^2 < y\}.$$

By Corollary 4.5, the probability for the existence of the ML estimate of $\boldsymbol{\zeta}$ in Ξ^* based on n observations is given by

$$(P_{\boldsymbol{\zeta}}^*)^{(n)}\left(\left\{(x_1, \ldots, x_n) \in \mathbb{R}^n : \frac{1}{n}\sum_{i=1}^{n} \boldsymbol{T}(x_i) \in \pi(\Xi^*)\right\}\right) = \begin{cases} 0, & n = 1, \\ 1, & n \geq 2, \end{cases}$$

since $(x_1, x_1^2)^t \notin \pi(\Xi^*)$ for all $x_1 \in \mathbb{R}$, and

$$\left(\frac{1}{n}\sum_{i=1}^{n} x_i\right)^2 \leq \frac{1}{n}\sum_{i=1}^{n} x_i^2$$

for all $x_1, \ldots, x_n \in \mathbb{R}$ and $n \geq 2$ (the empirical variance is non-negative) with equality if and only if $x_1 = \cdots = x_n$. Hence, for $n \geq 2$, the MLE of $\boldsymbol{\zeta}$ based on an iid sample $X_1, \ldots, X_n$ from P^*_ζ uniquely exists ($\mathbb{P}_\zeta$-a.s.) and is given by

$$\hat{\zeta}^{(n)} = \pi^{-1}\left(\frac{1}{n}\sum_{i=1}^{n} X_i, \frac{1}{n}\sum_{i=1}^{n} X_i^2\right)$$

with inverse function π^{-1} as stated in Example 2.59.

Example 4.10 From Example 2.65 for $\mathcal{P} = \mathcal{N}_k(\bullet, \boldsymbol{\Sigma}_0)$, we have $\boldsymbol{T}(\boldsymbol{x}) = \boldsymbol{\Sigma}_0^{-1}\boldsymbol{x}$ for $\boldsymbol{x} \in \mathbb{R}^k$, $\Xi^* = \mathbb{R}^k$, and $\pi(\boldsymbol{\mu}) = \boldsymbol{\Sigma}_0^{-1}\boldsymbol{\mu}$ for $\boldsymbol{\mu} \in \mathbb{R}^k$. Here, $\pi(\Xi^*) = \mathbb{R}^k$ such that condition (4.2) is trivially met. Hence, by Corollary 4.5, the MLE of $\boldsymbol{\mu}$ based on an iid sample $\boldsymbol{X}^{(1)}, \ldots, \boldsymbol{X}^{(n)}$ from $P_{\boldsymbol{\mu}}$ uniquely exists and is given by

$$\hat{\boldsymbol{\mu}}^{(n)} = \pi^{-1}\left(\frac{1}{n}\sum_{i=1}^{n} \boldsymbol{T}(\boldsymbol{X}^{(i)})\right) = \boldsymbol{\Sigma}_0\left(\frac{1}{n}\sum_{i=1}^{n} \boldsymbol{\Sigma}_0^{-1}\boldsymbol{X}^{(i)}\right) = \frac{1}{n}\sum_{i=1}^{n} \boldsymbol{X}^{(i)}.$$

4.2 Constrained Maximum Likelihood Estimation

We now consider maximum likelihood estimation in non-full EFs. Any such non-full family is represented by a subfamily $\{P^*_\zeta : \zeta \in \Xi\}$ of the full family $\{P^*_\zeta : \zeta \in \Xi^*\}$ for some proper subset Ξ of Ξ^* (with $\Xi \neq \Xi^*$). Thus, the aim is now to find all parameters within the *constrained* set Ξ at which the likelihood function has a global maximum on Ξ.

For every $x \in \mathcal{X}$ and every compact set $\Xi \subset int(\Xi^*)$, it is clear that there exists an ML estimate of ζ in Ξ based on x, since $\ell(\cdot; x)$ is continuous on Ξ by Lemma 4.2 and thus attains its maximum on Ξ. On the other hand, the strict concavity of $\ell(\cdot; x)$ on Ξ^* ensures uniqueness of the ML estimate in every convex set $\Xi \subset \Xi^*$ provided that it exists. Moreover, in the steep EF and if $\boldsymbol{T}(x) \in \pi(\Xi)$, then $\pi^{-1}(\boldsymbol{T}(x))$ must be the ML estimate in Ξ, since it already maximizes $\ell(\cdot; x)$ over Ξ^*. In [20, pp. 152–155], under different assumptions on the constrained set Ξ, sufficient and necessary conditions for the existence and uniqueness of ML estimates in non-full EFs are stated. The findings are presented in this section. First, as a preliminary result, we address the following lemma.

Lemma 4.11 *Let $\mathcal{P}$ be a full EF with minimal canonical representation (4.1). Moreover, let $x \in \mathcal{X}$ and $\emptyset \neq A \subset \mathbb{R}^k$ be closed. If*

$$\ell(\zeta) = \ell(\zeta; x) \to -\infty \quad \text{for } ||\zeta||_2 \to \infty, \tag{4.4}$$

then there exists some $\eta \in A$ with $\ell(\eta) = \sup_{\zeta \in A} \ell(\zeta)$.

Proof Let $m = \sup_{\boldsymbol{\zeta}\in A} \ell(\boldsymbol{\zeta})$, and $\boldsymbol{\zeta}_n \in A$, $n \in \mathbb{N}$, be a sequence with $\ell(\boldsymbol{\zeta}_n) \to m$ for $n \to \infty$. If $m = -\infty$, the assertion is trivially met. For $m > -\infty$, it holds by assumption that $\boldsymbol{\zeta}_n$, $n \in \mathbb{N}$, is bounded. Hence, there exists a convergent subsequence $\boldsymbol{\zeta}_{n_k}$, $k \in \mathbb{N}$, with $\boldsymbol{\zeta}_{n_k} \to \boldsymbol{\eta} \in A$ for $k \to \infty$. By Lemma 4.2, ℓ is upper semi-continuous, which yields

$$m \geq \ell(\boldsymbol{\eta}) \geq \limsup_{k\to\infty} \ell(\boldsymbol{\zeta}_{n_k}) = m\,,$$

i.e., $\ell(\boldsymbol{\eta}) = m$. □

To obtain a sufficient condition for property (4.4) to hold true, we introduce the half spaces

$$H^+(\boldsymbol{y}, a) = \{\boldsymbol{z} \in \mathbb{R}^k : \boldsymbol{y}^t\boldsymbol{z} > a\}\,,$$

$$H^-(\boldsymbol{y}, a) = \{\boldsymbol{z} \in \mathbb{R}^k : \boldsymbol{y}^t\boldsymbol{z} < a\}\,,$$

for $\boldsymbol{y} \in \mathbb{R}^k$ and $a \in \mathbb{R}$.

Lemma 4.12 *Let $\mathcal{P}$ be a full EF with minimal canonical representation (4.1), and let $\mathbf{0} \in int(M)$. Then, $\kappa(\boldsymbol{\zeta}) \to \infty$ for $||\boldsymbol{\zeta}||_2 \to \infty$.*

Proof First, we show that there exist some $a > 0$ and $c > 0$ such that

$$\nu^{\boldsymbol{T}}(H^+(\boldsymbol{y}, a)) > c \qquad \text{for all } \boldsymbol{y} \in B = \{\boldsymbol{z} \in \mathbb{R}^k : ||\boldsymbol{z}||_2 = 1\}\,.$$

Suppose the contrary assertion is true. Then, there exist a sequence a_n, $n \in \mathbb{N}$, with $\lim_{n\to\infty} a_n = 0$, and a sequence $\boldsymbol{y}_n \in B$, $n \in \mathbb{N}$, with

$$\lim_{n\to\infty} \nu^{\boldsymbol{T}}(H^+(\boldsymbol{y}_n, a_n)) = 0\,.$$

Since B is compact, there exist $\boldsymbol{y} \in B$ and a convergent subsequence $\boldsymbol{y}_{n_k}$, $k \in \mathbb{N}$, with $\boldsymbol{y}_{n_k} \to \boldsymbol{y}$ for $k \to \infty$. Note that, for every $\boldsymbol{z} \in \mathbb{R}^k$ with $\boldsymbol{y}^t\boldsymbol{z} > 0$, there exists an index $k_0 \in \mathbb{N}$ such that $\boldsymbol{y}_{n_k}^t\boldsymbol{z} > a_{n_k}$ for all $k \geq k_0$. Together with Fatou's lemma (see, e.g., [17, p. 209]), this yields

$$\begin{aligned}\nu^{\boldsymbol{T}}(H^+(\boldsymbol{y}, 0)) &= \int \mathbb{1}_{H^+(\boldsymbol{y},0)}\, d\nu^{\boldsymbol{T}} \leq \int \liminf_{k\to\infty} \mathbb{1}_{H^+(\boldsymbol{y}_{n_k}, a_{n_k})}\, d\nu^{\boldsymbol{T}} \\ &\leq \liminf_{k\to\infty} \int \mathbb{1}_{H^+(\boldsymbol{y}_{n_k}, a_{n_k})}\, d\nu^{\boldsymbol{T}} = \lim_{k\to\infty} \nu^{\boldsymbol{T}}(H^+(\boldsymbol{y}_{n_k}, a_{n_k})) = 0\,.\end{aligned}$$

Hence, we have $supp(\nu^{\boldsymbol{T}}) \subset H^+(\boldsymbol{y}, 0)^c$ and thus $M \subset H^+(\boldsymbol{y}, 0)^c$, since $H^+(\boldsymbol{y}, 0)^c$ is convex and closed. By assumption, $\mathbf{0} \in int(M)$, which gives the contradiction $\mathbf{0} \in int(H^+(\boldsymbol{y}, 0)^c) = H^-(\boldsymbol{y}, 0)$.

Now, for $\boldsymbol{\zeta} \in \mathbb{R}^k \setminus \{\mathbf{0}\}$,

$$\begin{aligned}\kappa(\boldsymbol{\zeta}) &= \ln\left(\int e^{\boldsymbol{\zeta}^t \boldsymbol{t}}\, d\nu^{\boldsymbol{T}}(\boldsymbol{t})\right) = \ln\left(\int \exp\left\{||\boldsymbol{\zeta}||_2 \left(\frac{\boldsymbol{\zeta}}{||\boldsymbol{\zeta}||_2}\right)^t \boldsymbol{t}\right\} d\nu^{\boldsymbol{T}}(\boldsymbol{t})\right)\\ &\geq \ln\left(\int_{H^+(\boldsymbol{\zeta}/||\boldsymbol{\zeta}||_2, a)} \exp\left\{||\boldsymbol{\zeta}||_2 \left(\frac{\boldsymbol{\zeta}}{||\boldsymbol{\zeta}||_2}\right)^t \boldsymbol{t}\right\} d\nu^{\boldsymbol{T}}(\boldsymbol{t})\right)\\ &\geq \ln\left(e^{||\boldsymbol{\zeta}||_2\, a}\, c\right) = a\, ||\boldsymbol{\zeta}||_2 + \ln(c)\,.\end{aligned}$$

For $||\boldsymbol{\zeta}||_2 \to \infty$, this yields the assertion. □

For a relatively closed subset Ξ of Ξ^*, we have the following theorem (see [20, pp. 152/153]).

Theorem 4.13 *Let $\mathcal{P}$ be a steep EF with minimal canonical representation (4.1), and let $x \in \mathcal{X}$ be a realization of the random variable X with distribution $P^*_{\boldsymbol{\zeta}} \in \mathcal{P}$. Moreover, let $\Xi \neq \emptyset$ be relatively closed in Ξ^*, i.e., $\Xi = B \cap \Xi^*$ for a closed set $B \subset \mathbb{R}^k$. Then, an ML estimate of $\boldsymbol{\zeta}$ in Ξ based on x exists if one of the following conditions is met:*

(a) $\boldsymbol{T}(x) \in int(M)$,

(b) $\boldsymbol{T}(x) \in M \setminus int(M)$ *and there exist* $\boldsymbol{t}_1, \ldots, \boldsymbol{t}_m \in int(M)$ *and* $a_1, \ldots, a_m \in \mathbb{R}$ *with*

$$\Xi \subset \bigcup_{i=1}^{m} H^-(\boldsymbol{T}(x) - \boldsymbol{t}_i, a_i)\,. \tag{4.5}$$

Proof Let $\boldsymbol{t} = \boldsymbol{T}(x)$. First, let (a) be true, i.e., $\boldsymbol{t} \in int(M)$. Since for $\boldsymbol{\zeta} \in \Xi^*$

$$f^*_{\boldsymbol{\zeta}} = e^{\boldsymbol{\zeta}^t \boldsymbol{T} - \kappa(\boldsymbol{\zeta})} h = e^{\boldsymbol{\zeta}^t(\boldsymbol{T}-\boldsymbol{t}) - (\kappa(\boldsymbol{\zeta}) - \boldsymbol{\zeta}^t \boldsymbol{t})} h$$

we have another representation of $\mathcal{P}$ with statistic $\check{\boldsymbol{T}} = \boldsymbol{T} - \boldsymbol{t}$ and cumulant function $\check{\kappa}(\boldsymbol{\zeta}) = \kappa(\boldsymbol{\zeta}) - \boldsymbol{\zeta}^t \boldsymbol{t}$, $\boldsymbol{\zeta} \in \mathbb{R}^k$. The corresponding convex support $\check{M}$ of $\nu^{\check{\boldsymbol{T}}}$ is then

$$\check{M} = M - \boldsymbol{t}$$

and satisfies $\mathbf{0} \in int(\check{M})$ by assumption. Hence, by Lemma 4.12, we have

$$\ell(\boldsymbol{\zeta}; x) = \ln(h(x)) - \check{\kappa}(\boldsymbol{\zeta}) \to -\infty$$

for $||\boldsymbol{\zeta}||_2 \to \infty$. Applying Lemma 4.11 then yields that there exists some $\boldsymbol{\eta} \in B$ with $\ell(\boldsymbol{\eta}; x) = \sup_{\boldsymbol{\zeta} \in B} \ell(\boldsymbol{\zeta}; x)$. Necessarily holds that $\boldsymbol{\eta} \in \Xi = B \cap \Xi^*$, since $\boldsymbol{\eta} \notin \Xi^*$ would imply that $\ell(\boldsymbol{\eta}; x) = -\infty$, which forms a contradiction to $\emptyset \neq \Xi \subset \Xi^*$.

Now, let assertion (b) be true. Since $\boldsymbol{t}_1, \ldots, \boldsymbol{t}_m \in int(M)$, we have $\kappa_i(\boldsymbol{\zeta}) = \kappa(\boldsymbol{\zeta}) - \boldsymbol{\zeta}^t \boldsymbol{t}_i \to \infty$ for $||\boldsymbol{\zeta}||_2 \to \infty$ and $1 \le i \le m$ by the same arguments as above. Moreover, for $\boldsymbol{\zeta} \in \Xi$, there exists an index $j \in \{1, \ldots, m\}$ with

$$\begin{aligned} \ell(\boldsymbol{\zeta}; x) &= \ln(h(x)) + \boldsymbol{\zeta}^t(\boldsymbol{T}(x) - \boldsymbol{t}_j) - \kappa_j(\boldsymbol{\zeta}) \\ &\le \ln(h(x)) + a_j - \kappa_j(\boldsymbol{\zeta}) . \end{aligned}$$

Thus,

$$\ell(\boldsymbol{\zeta}; x) \le \sup_{1 \le i \le m} \{\ln(h(x)) + a_i - \kappa_i(\boldsymbol{\zeta})\} \to -\infty$$

for $||\boldsymbol{\zeta}||_2 \to \infty$. Again, applying Lemma 4.11 completes the proof. □

Theorem 4.13 may be useful to ensure existence of ML estimates in curved EFs as indicated in the following remark.

Remark 4.14 Let $\mathcal{P}$ be a steep EF with minimal canonical representation (4.1). Moreover, let $\Theta \subset \mathbb{R}^m$ for some $m < k$,

$$\boldsymbol{Z} = (Z_1, \ldots, Z_k)^t : \quad \Theta \to \Xi^*$$

be a one-to-one mapping with $int(\boldsymbol{Z}(\Theta)) = \emptyset$, and $Z_1, \ldots, Z_K$ be affinely independent. Then, the non-full subfamily

$$\mathcal{P}_{\boldsymbol{Z}} = \{P^*_{\boldsymbol{Z}(\vartheta)} : \vartheta \in \Theta\}$$

of $\mathcal{P}$ forms a curved EF according to Definition 2.32. Now, let x be a realization of $X \sim P^*_{\boldsymbol{Z}(\vartheta)} \in \mathcal{P}_{\boldsymbol{Z}}$. If $\boldsymbol{Z}(\Theta)$ is relatively closed in Ξ^*, Theorem 4.13 is applicable and may be used to ensure existence of ML estimates of ϑ in Θ based on x. For example, an ML estimate of ϑ in Θ exists with probability 1 if the distribution of $\boldsymbol{T}$ has a Lebesgue density (see Remark 4.4). Under the additional assumptions that Θ is open, $\boldsymbol{Z}(\Theta) \subset int(\Xi^*)$, and $\boldsymbol{Z}$ is differentiable, any ML estimate of ϑ in Θ based on x is necessarily a solution of the likelihood equation

$$\mathbf{D}_{\boldsymbol{Z}}(\vartheta)^t \, [\boldsymbol{T}(x) - \pi(\boldsymbol{Z}(\vartheta))] = \mathbf{0} \tag{4.6}$$

with respect to $\vartheta \in \Theta$ (see Theorem 2.56). Note, however, that the likelihood function may have several local maxima and thus Eq. (4.6) more than one solution in Θ (see [5, p. 69]).

Uniqueness of the ML estimate may also be guaranteed by imposing further assumptions on both $\boldsymbol{Z}$ and $\boldsymbol{T}$. For instance, in case of Lebesgue density functions, the MLE of ϑ in Θ is unique with probability 1 if $\mathcal{X} \subset \mathbb{R}^n$ for some $n \ge k$ and $\mathcal{X}$ is open, Θ is open with $\boldsymbol{Z}(\Theta) \subset int(\Xi^*)$, $\boldsymbol{T}$ is continuously differentiable and $\boldsymbol{Z}$ is twice continuously differentiable with Jacobian matrix $\mathbf{D}_{\boldsymbol{T}}(x)$ of full rank k at every

$x \in \mathcal{X}$ and Jacobian matrix $\mathbf{D}_{\mathbf{Z}}(\vartheta)$ of full rank m at every $\vartheta \in \Theta$, respectively (see [49] and [38]).

Example: Curved EF in $\mathcal{N}(\bullet, \bullet)$

Example 4.15 We consider the curved EF $\mathcal{P}_2 = \{\mathcal{N}(\mu, \mu^2) : \mu \in \mathbb{R} \setminus \{0\}\}$ in Example 2.31(b) forming a subfamily of $\mathcal{N}(\bullet, \bullet)$ with $ord(\mathcal{P}_2) = 2$. By using the canonical representation of $\mathcal{N}(\bullet, \bullet)$ introduced in Example 2.39, we have $\mathcal{P}_2 = \{P^*_{\mathbf{Z}(\mu)} : \mu \in \Theta\}$ with $\Theta = \mathbb{R}\setminus\{0\}$ and $\mathbf{Z} = (Z_1, Z_2)^t : \Theta \to \Xi^* = \mathbb{R}\times(-\infty, 0)$, where

$$Z_1(\mu) = \frac{1}{\mu} \qquad \text{and} \qquad Z_2(\mu) = -\frac{1}{2\mu^2} \qquad \text{for } \mu \in \Theta\,.$$

The corresponding statistic is given by $\boldsymbol{T}(x) = (x, x^2)^t$, $x \in \mathbb{R}$. Obviously, $\mathbf{Z}$ is one-to-one, and

$$\mathbf{Z}(\Theta) = \{(\eta, -\eta^2/2)^t : \eta \in \mathbb{R} \setminus \{0\}\}$$

is relatively closed in Ξ^*, since $\mathbf{Z}(\Theta) = B \cap \Xi^*$ for $B = \{(\eta, -\eta^2/2)^t : \eta \in \mathbb{R}\}$, which is closed in $\mathbb{R}^2$. From Remark 2.62 and Example 2.59, we have that

$$int(M) = \pi(\Xi^*) = \{(x, y)^t \in \mathbb{R}^2 : x^2 < y\}\,.$$

Now, let us assume to have realizations $x_1, \ldots, x_n$ of an iid sample $X_1, \ldots, X_n$ of size $n \geq 2$ from $P^*_{\mathbf{Z}(\mu)}$ for some $\mu \in \Theta$. Since

$$\frac{1}{n}\sum_{i=1}^{n} \boldsymbol{T}(x_i) = \left(\frac{1}{n}\sum_{i=1}^{n} x_i\,,\ \frac{1}{n}\sum_{i=1}^{n} x_i^2\right)^t \in int(M)$$

if $x_1, \ldots, x_n$ are not all identical (see Example 4.9), Theorem 4.13 applied to the product EF $\mathcal{P}^{(n)}$ with statistic $\boldsymbol{T}^{(n)}(\boldsymbol{x}) = \sum_{i=1}^n \boldsymbol{T}(x_i)$ for $\boldsymbol{x} = (x_1, \ldots, x_n) \in \mathcal{X}^n = \mathbb{R}^n$ ensures that an MLE of μ in Θ based on $X_1, \ldots, X_n$ exists with probability 1. Moreover, the MLE is uniquely determined with probability 1 by Remark 4.14. To see this, we formally replace the sample space $\mathcal{X}^n = \mathbb{R}^n$ by $\mathcal{Y} = \mathbb{R}^n \setminus N$, where $N = \{(x, \ldots, x) \in \mathbb{R}^n : x \in \mathbb{R}\}$ has probability 0. Then, $\mathcal{Y}$ is open and $\boldsymbol{T}^{(n)}$ is continuously differentiable on $\mathcal{Y}$ with Jacobian matrix

$$\mathbf{D}_{\boldsymbol{T}^{(n)}}(\boldsymbol{y}) = \begin{pmatrix} \mathbf{1} \\ 2\boldsymbol{y} \end{pmatrix}, \qquad \boldsymbol{y} \in \mathcal{Y}\,,$$

with $\mathbf{1} = (1, \ldots, 1) \in \mathbb{R}^n$, which has full rank $k = 2 \leq n$ at every $\boldsymbol{y} \in \mathcal{Y}$. Since $\Theta = \mathbb{R} \setminus \{0\}$ is open and $\boldsymbol{Z}$ is twice continuously differentiable with Jacobian matrix

$$\mathbf{D}_{\boldsymbol{Z}}(\mu) = \left(-\frac{1}{\mu^2}, \frac{1}{\mu^3}\right)^t$$

of rank $m = 1$ at every $\mu \in \Theta$, all conditions in Remark 4.14 for the uniqueness of the MLE are met (see also [49, Ex. 3]).

If Ξ in Theorem 4.13 is moreover convex, the ML estimate of $\boldsymbol{\zeta}$ in Ξ based on x is unique provided that it exists. Furthermore, we have the following theorem (see [20, pp. 153–155]).

Theorem 4.16 *In the situation of Theorem 4.13, let Ξ be moreover convex and $\Xi \cap int(\Xi^*) \neq \emptyset$. Then, there exists a unique ML estimate of $\boldsymbol{\zeta}$ in Ξ based on x if and only if one of the following conditions is met:*

(a) $\boldsymbol{T}(x) \in int(M)$,
(b) $\boldsymbol{T}(x) \in M \setminus int(M)$ *and there exist* $\boldsymbol{t}_1 \in int(M)$ *and* $a_1 \in \mathbb{R}$ *with*

$$\Xi \subset H^-(\boldsymbol{T}(x) - \boldsymbol{t}_1, a_1) .$$

If an ML estimate of $\boldsymbol{\zeta}$ in Ξ based on x exists, it is the unique parameter $\boldsymbol{\zeta}^* \in \Xi \cap int(\Xi^*)$ satisfying

$$(\boldsymbol{T}(x) - \pi(\boldsymbol{\zeta}^*))^t(\boldsymbol{\zeta}^* - \boldsymbol{\eta}) \geq 0 \qquad \text{for all } \boldsymbol{\eta} \in \Xi . \tag{4.7}$$

Proof First, let us show that if inequality (4.7) has a solution in $\Xi \cap int(\Xi^*)$, it is uniquely determined. For this, let $\boldsymbol{\zeta}_1^*, \boldsymbol{\zeta}_2^* \in \Xi \cap int(\Xi^*)$ be solutions of inequality (4.7). Then, in particular,

$$(\boldsymbol{T}(x) - \pi(\boldsymbol{\zeta}_1^*))^t(\boldsymbol{\zeta}_1^* - \boldsymbol{\zeta}_2^*) \geq 0 ,$$

$$(\boldsymbol{T}(x) - \pi(\boldsymbol{\zeta}_2^*))^t(\boldsymbol{\zeta}_2^* - \boldsymbol{\zeta}_1^*) \geq 0 .$$

Summation of both inequalities and applying Lemma 3.37 yields

$$0 \leq (\pi(\boldsymbol{\zeta}_2^*) - \pi(\boldsymbol{\zeta}_1^*))^t(\boldsymbol{\zeta}_1^* - \boldsymbol{\zeta}_2^*) = -D_J(\boldsymbol{\zeta}_1^*, \boldsymbol{\zeta}_2^*)$$

By Remark 3.40, it follows that $D_J(\boldsymbol{\zeta}_1^*, \boldsymbol{\zeta}_2^*) = 0$ and $\boldsymbol{\zeta}_1^* = \boldsymbol{\zeta}_2^*$.

Next, let us show that $\boldsymbol{\zeta}^*$ is an ML estimate of $\boldsymbol{\zeta}$ in Ξ based on x if and only if $\boldsymbol{\zeta}^* \in \Xi \cap int(\Xi^*)$ and $\boldsymbol{\zeta}^*$ satisfies inequality (4.7).

First, if $\boldsymbol{\zeta}^* \notin \Xi \cap int(\Xi^*)$, $\boldsymbol{\zeta}$ cannot be an ML estimate of $\boldsymbol{\zeta}$ in Ξ based on x, since the steepness of $\mathcal{P}$ ensures the existence of some $\boldsymbol{\eta} \in \Xi \cap int(\Xi^*)$ with $\ell(\boldsymbol{\eta}; x) > \ell(\boldsymbol{\zeta}; x)$, as shown in the proof of Theorem 4.3. Now, let $\boldsymbol{\zeta}^* \in \Xi \cap int(\Xi^*)$ and suppose that there exists some $\boldsymbol{\eta} \in \Xi$ with

$$(\boldsymbol{T}(x) - \pi(\boldsymbol{\zeta}^*))^t(\boldsymbol{\zeta}^* - \boldsymbol{\eta}) < 0 .$$

Since Ξ is convex by assumption, $\boldsymbol{\eta}^{(\alpha)} = \boldsymbol{\zeta}^* + \alpha(\boldsymbol{\eta} - \boldsymbol{\zeta}^*) \in \Xi$, $\alpha \in [0, 1]$, and we obtain from Lemma 4.2

$$\frac{\partial}{\partial \alpha} \ell(\boldsymbol{\eta}^{(\alpha)}; x)\bigg|_{\alpha=0} = (\boldsymbol{T}(x) - \pi(\boldsymbol{\zeta}^*))^t(\boldsymbol{\eta} - \boldsymbol{\zeta}^*) > 0 .$$

Hence, there exists $\tilde{\alpha} \in (0, 1)$ with $\ell(\boldsymbol{\eta}^{(\tilde{\alpha})}; x) > \ell(\boldsymbol{\zeta}^*; x)$, which implies that $\boldsymbol{\zeta}^*$ is not an ML estimate of $\boldsymbol{\zeta}$ in Ξ based on x.

Now, let $\boldsymbol{\zeta}^* \in \Xi \cap int(\Xi^*)$ satisfy inequality (4.7). Then, by using Lemma 3.37, it holds for $\boldsymbol{\eta} \in \Xi \cap int(\Xi^*)$ that

$$\begin{aligned} \ell(\boldsymbol{\zeta}^*; x) - \ell(\boldsymbol{\eta}; x) &= (\boldsymbol{\zeta}^* - \boldsymbol{\eta})^t \boldsymbol{T}(x) - \kappa(\boldsymbol{\zeta}^*) + \kappa(\boldsymbol{\eta}) \\ &= (\boldsymbol{\zeta}^* - \boldsymbol{\eta})^t (\boldsymbol{T}(x) - \pi(\boldsymbol{\zeta}^*)) + D_{KL}(\boldsymbol{\zeta}^*, \boldsymbol{\eta}) \\ &\geq 0 , \end{aligned}$$

since $\boldsymbol{\zeta}^*$ satisfies inequality (4.7) and D_{KL} is non-negative by Remark 3.40. Moreover, by the same arguments as in the proof of Theorem 4.3, the steepness of $\mathcal{P}$ ensures that for every $\tilde{\boldsymbol{\eta}} \in \Xi \cap (\Xi^* \setminus int(\Xi^*))$ there exists some $\boldsymbol{\eta} \in \Xi \cap int(\Xi^*)$ with $\ell(\boldsymbol{\eta}; x) > \ell(\tilde{\boldsymbol{\eta}}; x)$. Hence, $\boldsymbol{\zeta}^*$ is an ML estimate of $\boldsymbol{\zeta}$ in Ξ based on x.

Finally, we prove the equivalence assertion. If either statement (a) or (b) is met, then existence of an ML estimate of $\boldsymbol{\zeta}$ in Ξ based on x follows from Theorem 4.13. Since $\ell(\cdot; x)$ is strictly concave on Ξ by Lemma 4.2, this ML estimate is uniquely determined. For the other implication, let $\boldsymbol{\zeta}^*$ denote the unique ML estimate of $\boldsymbol{\zeta}$ in Ξ based on x. Then, as already shown above, $\boldsymbol{\zeta}^* \in \Xi \cap int(\Xi^*)$ and $\boldsymbol{\zeta}^*$ satisfies inequality (4.7), which is equivalent to

$$\boldsymbol{\eta}^t(\boldsymbol{T}(x) - \pi(\boldsymbol{\zeta}^*)) \leq (\boldsymbol{\zeta}^*)^t(\boldsymbol{T}(x) - \pi(\boldsymbol{\zeta}^*)) \qquad \text{for all } \boldsymbol{\eta} \in \Xi .$$

Hence, assertion (b) is true with $\boldsymbol{t}_1 = \pi(\boldsymbol{\zeta}^*) \in int(M)$ and some arbitrary $a_1 > (\boldsymbol{\zeta}^*)^t(\boldsymbol{T}(x) - \pi(\boldsymbol{\zeta}^*))$. □

For more details on maximum likelihood estimation in EFs including, in particular, geometrical interpretations and illustrations of formulas (4.5) and (4.7), see [20, Chapter 5].

So far in this chapter, we have considered maximum likelihood estimation for the natural parameter of the EF. For the sake of completeness, we finally address a result and a comment for other parametrizations.

Lemma 4.17 *Let $\mathcal{P}$ be an EF with minimal canonical representation (4.1). Moreover, let $\Delta \subset \mathbb{R}^k$, $\Psi : \Delta \to \Xi$ be a bijective mapping, and $\tilde{P}_\eta = P^*_{\Psi(\eta)}$, $\eta \in \Delta$, denote the corresponding parametrization of $\mathcal{P}$ with μ-density $\tilde{f}_\eta = f^*_{\Psi(\eta)}$ of $\tilde{P}_\eta$ for $\eta \in \Delta$. Let x be a realization of the random variable X with distribution in $\mathcal{P}$, and let $\check{\boldsymbol{\zeta}}$ denote an ML estimate of $\boldsymbol{\zeta}$ in Ξ based on x. Then, $\check{\eta} = \Psi^{-1}(\check{\boldsymbol{\zeta}})$ is an ML estimate of η in Δ based on x. Moreover, if $\check{\boldsymbol{\zeta}}$ is uniquely determined, so is $\check{\eta}$.*

Proof Since Ψ is bijective, we have

$$\tilde{f}_{\Psi^{-1}(\check{\boldsymbol{\zeta}})}(x) \geq \tilde{f}_\eta(x) \quad \text{for all } \eta \in \Delta \qquad \Leftrightarrow \qquad f^*_{\check{\boldsymbol{\zeta}}}(x) \geq f^*_{\Psi(\eta)}(x) \quad \text{for all } \eta \in \Delta$$

$$\Leftrightarrow \qquad f^*_{\check{\boldsymbol{\zeta}}}(x) \geq f^*_{\boldsymbol{\zeta}}(x) \quad \text{for all } \boldsymbol{\zeta} \in \Xi\,,$$

which is true by assumption. Hence, $\check{\eta} = \Psi^{-1}(\check{\boldsymbol{\zeta}})$ is an ML estimate of η in Δ based on x. If $\check{\boldsymbol{\zeta}}$ is uniquely determined, then the above equivalences hold true with strict inequalities when replacing Δ by $\Delta \setminus \{\check{\eta}\}$ and Ξ by $\Xi \setminus \{\check{\boldsymbol{\zeta}}\}$, and $\check{\eta}$ is uniquely determined as well. □

Simply put, Lemma 4.17 states that an ML estimate for a (bijectively) transformed parameter can be obtained by transforming an ML estimate for the original parameter in the same way. This property holds true in parametric models, in general.

From Lemma 4.17, respective statements for the iid case and for the existence and uniqueness of the MLE of η can readily be deduced. As an important example for minimal regular EFs, these results apply to the mean value parametrization $\tilde{P}_{\boldsymbol{m}}$, $\boldsymbol{m} \in int(M)$, by setting $\Psi = \pi^{-1}$ (see Theorem 2.56). For instance, provided that the MLE $\hat{\boldsymbol{\zeta}}^{(n)}$ of $\boldsymbol{\zeta}$ in Ξ^* based on an iid sample $X^{(1)}, \ldots, X^{(n)}$ from $P^*_{\boldsymbol{\zeta}}$ exists, the MLE of $\boldsymbol{m}$ in $int(M)$ based on $X^{(1)}, \ldots, X^{(n)}$ is given by

$$\hat{\boldsymbol{m}}^{(n)} = \pi(\hat{\boldsymbol{\zeta}}^{(n)}) = \frac{1}{n}\sum_{i=1}^{n} \boldsymbol{T}(X^{(i)})\,,$$

where we still use the representation of $\hat{\boldsymbol{\zeta}}^{(n)}$ in Definition 4.6.

4.3 Efficient Estimation

We now turn to properties of point estimators and their connections to EFs. First of all, unbiasedness of an estimator means that, in expectation, we estimate correctly.

Definition 4.18 Let $\gamma : \Xi \to \mathbb{R}^q$ be a function. An estimator $\hat{\gamma} : (\Omega, \mathcal{A}, \mathbb{P}_{\boldsymbol{\zeta}}) \to (\mathbb{R}^q, \mathbb{B}^q)$ is called *unbiased for* γ if

$$\mathbb{E}_{\boldsymbol{\zeta}}[\hat{\gamma}] = \gamma(\boldsymbol{\zeta}) \qquad \text{for every } \boldsymbol{\zeta} \in \Xi\,.$$

In particular, an estimator $\hat{\boldsymbol{\zeta}}$ is called *unbiased for* $\boldsymbol{\zeta}$ if

$$\mathbb{E}_{\boldsymbol{\zeta}}[\hat{\boldsymbol{\zeta}}] = \boldsymbol{\zeta} \qquad \text{for every } \boldsymbol{\zeta} \in \Xi\,.$$

Remark 4.19 If under the assumptions of Corollary 4.5 the MLE $\hat{\boldsymbol{\zeta}}^{(n)}$ in formula (4.3) exists with probability 1, it is a measurable function of the sufficient and complete statistic $\boldsymbol{T}^{(n)}$ (see Corollary 3.21 and Theorem 3.13). For the one-parameter EF, the Lehmann-Scheffé theorem then yields that any estimator $c\hat{\zeta}^{(n)}$ being unbiased for ζ for some constant $c \in \mathbb{R}$ has minimum variance among all unbiased estimators for ζ. In that case, $c\hat{\zeta}^{(n)}$ is called a *uniformly minimum variance unbiased estimator* (UMVUE) for ζ.

Estimators with such a minimality property may also be defined in the multivariate case. The *Cramér-Rao inequality* provides a lower bound for the covariance matrix of any unbiased estimator.

Theorem 4.20 *Let $\mathcal{P}$ be an EF with minimal canonical representation (4.1), $\Xi \subset \Xi^*$ be open, and $\gamma : \Xi \to \mathbb{R}^q$ be a differentiable function. Moreover, let X be a random variable with distribution $P^*_{\boldsymbol{\zeta}}$ for some $\boldsymbol{\zeta} \in \Xi$. Then, for every unbiased estimator $\hat{\gamma}$ for γ based on X, the Cramér-Rao inequality*

$$\mathbb{C}\mathrm{ov}_{\boldsymbol{\zeta}}(\hat{\gamma}) \geq \mathbf{D}_{\gamma}(\boldsymbol{\zeta})\,[\mathbf{I}(\boldsymbol{\zeta})]^{-1}\,\mathbf{D}_{\gamma}(\boldsymbol{\zeta})^t \tag{4.8}$$

holds true in the sense of the Löwner order for matrices defined by $\mathbf{A} \geq \mathbf{B}$ if and only if $\mathbf{A} - \mathbf{B} \geq 0$, i.e., $\mathbf{A} - \mathbf{B}$ is positive semidefinite. In particular, any unbiased estimator $\hat{\boldsymbol{\zeta}}$ for $\boldsymbol{\zeta}$ based on X satisfies that

$$\mathbb{C}\mathrm{ov}_{\boldsymbol{\zeta}}(\hat{\boldsymbol{\zeta}}) \geq [\mathbf{I}(\boldsymbol{\zeta})]^{-1}\,.$$

Here, $\mathbf{D}_{\gamma}(\boldsymbol{\zeta}) \in \mathbb{R}^{q \times k}$ denotes the Jacobian matrix of γ and $\mathbf{I}(\boldsymbol{\zeta})$ the Fisher information matrix of $\mathcal{P}$ at $\boldsymbol{\zeta}$.

Proof Let $\boldsymbol{\zeta} \in \Xi$. Note that then $\boldsymbol{\zeta} \in int(\Xi^*)$, since Ξ is open by assumption. Recall that by Theorems 3.29, 2.23, and Lemma 2.26

$$\boldsymbol{U}_{\boldsymbol{\zeta}} = \boldsymbol{T} - E_{\boldsymbol{\zeta}}[\boldsymbol{T}] \qquad \text{and} \qquad \mathbf{I}(\boldsymbol{\zeta}) = \mathbf{Cov}_{\boldsymbol{\zeta}}(\boldsymbol{T}) > 0\,.$$

In particular, we have

$$E_\zeta[\boldsymbol{U}_\zeta] = \mathbf{0} \qquad \text{and} \qquad \mathbf{Cov}_\zeta(\boldsymbol{U}_\zeta) = \mathbf{I}(\boldsymbol{\zeta})\,. \tag{4.9}$$

Since $\hat{\gamma} = (\hat{\gamma}_1, \ldots, \hat{\gamma}_q)^t$ is unbiased for $\gamma = (\gamma_1, \ldots, \gamma_q)^t$, Corollary 2.55 then yields for $1 \le j \le q$ that

$$\begin{aligned}\nabla\gamma_j(\boldsymbol{\zeta}) &= \nabla\mathbb{E}_\zeta[\hat{\gamma}_j] = \mathbb{C}\mathrm{ov}_\zeta(\hat{\gamma}_j, \boldsymbol{T}(X)) \\ &= \mathbb{C}\mathrm{ov}_\zeta(\hat{\gamma}_j, \boldsymbol{U}_\zeta(X)) = \mathbb{E}_\zeta[\hat{\gamma}_j\,\boldsymbol{U}_\zeta(X)]\,,\end{aligned}$$

i.e.,

$$\mathbf{D}_\gamma(\boldsymbol{\zeta}) = \mathbb{E}_\zeta[\hat{\gamma}\,\boldsymbol{U}_\zeta(X)^t]\,.$$

Now, for $\boldsymbol{y} \in \mathbb{R}^q$, it follows by inserting and by using formula (4.9) that

$$\begin{aligned}\boldsymbol{y}^t\,\mathbf{D}_\gamma(\boldsymbol{\zeta})\,[\mathbf{I}(\boldsymbol{\zeta})]^{-1}\,\mathbf{D}_\gamma(\boldsymbol{\zeta})^t\,\boldsymbol{y} &= \mathbb{E}_\zeta[\boldsymbol{y}^t\,\hat{\gamma}\,\boldsymbol{U}_\zeta(X)^t\,[\mathbf{I}(\boldsymbol{\zeta})]^{-1}\,\mathbf{D}_\gamma(\boldsymbol{\zeta})^t\,\boldsymbol{y}] \\ &= \mathbb{E}_\zeta[[\boldsymbol{y}^t\,(\hat{\gamma} - \gamma(\boldsymbol{\zeta}))]\,[\boldsymbol{U}_\zeta(X)^t\,[\mathbf{I}(\boldsymbol{\zeta})]^{-1}\,\mathbf{D}_\gamma(\boldsymbol{\zeta})^t\,\boldsymbol{y}]] \\ &= \mathbb{C}\mathrm{ov}_\zeta(\boldsymbol{y}^t\,(\hat{\gamma} - \gamma(\boldsymbol{\zeta}))\,,\;\boldsymbol{U}_\zeta(X)^t\,[\mathbf{I}(\boldsymbol{\zeta})]^{-1}\,\mathbf{D}_\gamma(\boldsymbol{\zeta})^t\,\boldsymbol{y}).\end{aligned}$$

From the unbiasedness of $\hat{\gamma}$ and formula (4.9), the last expression is seen to be the covariance of two random variables with mean 0. Applying the Cauchy-Schwarz inequality then leads to

$$\begin{aligned}&[\boldsymbol{y}^t\,\mathbf{D}_\gamma(\boldsymbol{\zeta})\,[\mathbf{I}(\boldsymbol{\zeta})]^{-1}\,\mathbf{D}_\gamma(\boldsymbol{\zeta})^t\,\boldsymbol{y}]^2 \\ &\le \mathbb{V}\mathrm{ar}_\zeta(\boldsymbol{y}^t\,(\hat{\gamma} - \gamma(\boldsymbol{\zeta})))\;\mathbb{V}\mathrm{ar}_\zeta(\boldsymbol{U}_\zeta(X)^t\,[\mathbf{I}(\boldsymbol{\zeta})]^{-1}\,\mathbf{D}_\gamma(\boldsymbol{\zeta})^t\,\boldsymbol{y}) \\ &= [\boldsymbol{y}^t\,\mathbb{C}\mathrm{ov}_\zeta(\hat{\gamma})\,\boldsymbol{y}]\,[\boldsymbol{y}^t\,\mathbf{D}_\gamma(\boldsymbol{\zeta})\,[\mathbf{I}(\boldsymbol{\zeta})]^{-1}\,\mathbb{C}\mathrm{ov}_\zeta(\boldsymbol{U}_\zeta(X))\,[\mathbf{I}(\boldsymbol{\zeta})]^{-1}\,\mathbf{D}_\gamma(\boldsymbol{\zeta})^t\,\boldsymbol{y}] \\ &= [\boldsymbol{y}^t\,\mathbb{C}\mathrm{ov}_\zeta(\hat{\gamma})\,\boldsymbol{y}]\,[\boldsymbol{y}^t\,\mathbf{D}_\gamma(\boldsymbol{\zeta})\,[\mathbf{I}(\boldsymbol{\zeta})]^{-1}\,\mathbf{D}_\gamma(\boldsymbol{\zeta})^t\,\boldsymbol{y}]\,.\end{aligned}$$

Hence,

$$\boldsymbol{y}^t\,\mathbf{D}_\gamma(\boldsymbol{\zeta})\,[\mathbf{I}(\boldsymbol{\zeta})]^{-1}\,\mathbf{D}_\gamma(\boldsymbol{\zeta})^t\,\boldsymbol{y} \le \boldsymbol{y}^t\,\mathbb{C}\mathrm{ov}_\zeta(\hat{\gamma})\,\boldsymbol{y}\,,$$

which yields the assertion. □

Note that in the proof of Theorem 4.20 we use properties of the EF but not the explicit structure of the densities. Under respective assumptions such as those in formula (4.9), the Cramér-Rao inequality can be shown to hold true in more general models.

Efficient estimators are now introduced as follows, where we implicitly assume that the Cramér-Rao inequality is valid.

Definition 4.21 Let $\Xi \subset \Xi^*$ be open, $\gamma : \Xi \to \mathbb{R}^q$ be a differentiable function, and $\hat{\gamma} : (\Omega, \mathcal{A}, \mathbb{P}_\zeta) \to (\mathbb{R}^q, \mathbb{B}^q)$ be an unbiased estimator for γ. Then, $\hat{\gamma}$ is called *efficient for* γ if its covariance matrix attains the lower bound of the Cramér-Rao inequality in formula (4.8) for every $\zeta \in \Xi$, i.e.,

$$\mathbb{C}\mathrm{ov}_\zeta(\hat{\gamma}) = \mathbf{D}_\gamma(\zeta)\,[\mathbf{I}(\zeta)]^{-1}\,\mathbf{D}_\gamma(\zeta)^t\,, \qquad \zeta \in \Xi\,.$$

In particular, any unbiased estimator $\hat{\zeta}$ for ζ with $\mathbb{C}\mathrm{ov}_\zeta(\hat{\zeta}) = [\mathbf{I}(\zeta)]^{-1}$, $\zeta \in \Xi$, is called *efficient for* ζ.

An efficient estimator in the sense of Definition 4.21 simultaneously solves different optimization problems.

Remark 4.22 Let $\mathbf{A} = [a_{ij}]_{1\le i,j\le k}$, $\mathbf{B} = [b_{ij}]_{1\le i,j\le k} \in \mathbb{R}^{k\times k}$ be two matrices with $\mathbf{A}, \mathbf{B} \ge \mathbf{0}$ and $\mathbf{A} \ge \mathbf{B}$ in the sense of the Löwner order. Then,

(a) $a_{ii} \ge b_{ii}$, $1 \le i \le k$,
(b) trace($\mathbf{A}$) $\ge$ trace($\mathbf{B}$),
(c) det($\mathbf{A}$) $\ge$ det($\mathbf{B}$).

Note that (a) is obvious from $\boldsymbol{e}^t\mathbf{A}\boldsymbol{e} \ge \boldsymbol{e}^t\mathbf{B}\boldsymbol{e}$ for any unit vector $\boldsymbol{e} \in \mathbb{R}^k$, and (b) directly follows from (a); assertion (c) can be obtained from Weyl's Monotonicity Theorem stating that the j-th largest eigenvalue of $\mathbf{A}$ is not smaller than that of $\mathbf{B}$ for $1 \le j \le k$ if $\mathbf{A}, \mathbf{B} \ge 0$ and $\mathbf{A} - \mathbf{B} \ge 0$ (see [15, p. 63]). An efficient estimator therefore minimizes the marginal variances (a), the *total variation* (b), and the *generalized variance* (c) among all unbiased estimators. Here, the total variation and generalized variance of a random vector are defined as the trace and determinant of its covariance matrix, respectively (see, e.g., [45, p. 13 and pp. 30/31]).

Remark 4.23 For $k = 1$, an efficient estimator is always a UMVUE. The reverse implication is not true in general, since the lower bound of the Cramér-Rao inequality need not to be attained by the UMVUE. Indeed, it can be shown that efficient estimators essentially only exist in EFs (see, e.g., [16, pp. 182/183]). Analogously, for $k > 1$, efficiency of an estimator ensures that it has minimum covariance matrix in the sense of the Löwner order among all unbiased estimators, but not vice versa.

Examples: $\mathcal{G}(\bullet, \bullet)$, $\mathcal{N}_k(\bullet, \boldsymbol{\Sigma}_0)$

Example 4.24 Let $\mathcal{P} = \mathcal{G}(\bullet, \bullet)$ and $X_1, \ldots, X_n$ be an iid sample from $P_{\boldsymbol{\zeta}}^* \in \mathcal{P}$ (see Example 2.40). Evidently, $\sum_{i=1}^n X_i/n$ is an unbiased estimator for the mean $\mathbb{E}_{\boldsymbol{\zeta}}[X_1]$, which is given by $\pi_1(\boldsymbol{\zeta}) = -\zeta_2/\zeta_1$ in the natural parametrization as shown in Example 2.53. From Example 3.34, the Fisher information matrix of $\mathcal{P}^{(n)}$ is seen to be

$$n\mathbf{I}(\boldsymbol{\zeta}) = n\begin{pmatrix} \frac{\zeta_2}{\zeta_1^2} & -\frac{1}{\zeta_1} \\ -\frac{1}{\zeta_1} & \psi_1(\zeta_2) \end{pmatrix}, \qquad \boldsymbol{\zeta} = (\zeta_1, \zeta_2)^t \in (-\infty, 0) \times (0, \infty).$$

Hence, by setting $\gamma = \pi_1$, the lower bound of the Cramér-Rao inequality in formula (4.8) is obtained as

$$\left(\frac{\zeta_2}{\zeta_1^2}, -\frac{1}{\zeta_1}\right) \frac{1}{n\det(\mathbf{I}(\boldsymbol{\zeta}))} \begin{pmatrix} \psi_1(\zeta_2) & \frac{1}{\zeta_1} \\ \frac{1}{\zeta_1} & \frac{\zeta_2}{\zeta_1^2} \end{pmatrix} \begin{pmatrix} \frac{\zeta_2}{\zeta_1^2} \\ -\frac{1}{\zeta_1} \end{pmatrix}$$

$$= \frac{\zeta_1^2}{n(\zeta_2\Psi_1(\zeta_2) - 1)} \left(\frac{\zeta_2}{\zeta_1^2}, -\frac{1}{\zeta_1}\right) \begin{pmatrix} \frac{\zeta_2\Psi_1(\zeta_2)-1}{\zeta_1^2} \\ 0 \end{pmatrix} = \frac{\zeta_2}{n\zeta_1^2}$$

for $\boldsymbol{\zeta} = (\zeta_1, \zeta_2)^t \in (-\infty, 0) \times (0, \infty)$. From Example 2.53, we have $\mathbb{V}\mathrm{ar}_{\boldsymbol{\zeta}}(X_1) = \zeta_2/\zeta_1^2$ such that the variance of $\sum_{i=1}^n X_i/n$ attains the lower bound of the Cramér-Rao inequality. Thus, $\sum_{i=1}^n X_i/n$ is an efficient estimator (and a UMVUE) for π_1.

Example 4.25 Let $\mathcal{P} = \mathcal{N}_k(\bullet, \boldsymbol{\Sigma}_0)$ and $\boldsymbol{X}^{(1)}, \ldots, \boldsymbol{X}^{(n)}$ be an iid sample from $P_{\boldsymbol{\mu}} \in \mathcal{P}$. By Example 3.35, the Fisher information matrix of $\mathcal{P}^{(n)}$ is given by $n\boldsymbol{\Sigma}_0^{-1}$ at every $\boldsymbol{\mu} \in \mathbb{R}^k$. Accordingly, by Theorem 4.20, the covariance matrix of any unbiased estimator for $\boldsymbol{\mu}$ is bounded from below by $\boldsymbol{\Sigma}_0/n$. This is the covariance matrix of the MLE $\hat{\boldsymbol{\mu}}^{(n)} = \sum_{i=1}^n \boldsymbol{X}^{(i)}/n$ derived in Example 4.10, which is unbiased and therefore also efficient for $\boldsymbol{\mu}$.

Example 4.24 provides an efficient estimator for the mean of a gamma distribution. This finding is a particular case of a general result for EFs.

Theorem 4.26 *Let $\mathcal{P}$ be an EF with minimal canonical representation (4.1), $\Xi \subset \Xi^*$ be open, and X be a random variable with distribution in $\mathcal{P}$. Then, $\boldsymbol{T}(X)$ is an* *efficient estimator for $\pi(\boldsymbol{\zeta})$, $\boldsymbol{\zeta} \in \Xi$, where π is the mean value function as defined in Theorem 2.56.*

Proof Trivially, $\boldsymbol{T}(X)$ is an unbiased estimator for $\pi(\boldsymbol{\zeta}) = E_{\boldsymbol{\zeta}}[\boldsymbol{T}(X)]$, $\boldsymbol{\zeta} \in \Xi$. Moreover, from Theorems 2.56 and 3.29, we obtain that

$$\begin{aligned}\mathbf{D}_\pi(\boldsymbol{\zeta})\,[\mathbf{I}(\boldsymbol{\zeta})]^{-1}\,\mathbf{D}_\pi(\boldsymbol{\zeta})^t &= \mathbf{Cov}_{\boldsymbol{\zeta}}(\boldsymbol{T})\,[\mathbf{Cov}_{\boldsymbol{\zeta}}(\boldsymbol{T})]^{-1}\,\mathbf{Cov}_{\boldsymbol{\zeta}}(\boldsymbol{T}) \\ &= \mathbb{Cov}_{\boldsymbol{\zeta}}(\boldsymbol{T}(X)), \qquad \boldsymbol{\zeta} \in \Xi.\end{aligned}$$

□

Based on an iid sample, we arrive at the following version of Theorem 4.26.

Corollary 4.27 *Let $\mathcal{P}$ be an EF with minimal canonical representation (4.1), $\Xi \subset \Xi^*$ be open, and π be the corresponding mean value function as defined in Theorem 2.56. Moreover, let $X^{(1)}, \ldots, X^{(n)}$ be an iid sample from a distribution in $\mathcal{P}$. Then, $\sum_{i=1}^n \boldsymbol{T}(X^{(i)})/n$ is an efficient estimator for $\pi(\boldsymbol{\zeta})$, $\boldsymbol{\zeta} \in \Xi$.*

Proof Since $n\mathbf{I}(\boldsymbol{\zeta})$ is the Fisher information matrix of the product EF $\mathcal{P}^{(n)}$ at $\boldsymbol{\zeta}$, the lower bound of the Cramér-Rao inequality is here

$$\begin{aligned}\mathbf{D}_\pi(\boldsymbol{\zeta})\,[n\mathbf{I}(\boldsymbol{\zeta})]^{-1}\,\mathbf{D}_\pi(\boldsymbol{\zeta})^t &= \frac{\mathbb{Cov}_{\boldsymbol{\zeta}}(\boldsymbol{T}(X^{(1)}))}{n} \\ &= \mathbb{Cov}_{\boldsymbol{\zeta}}\left(\frac{1}{n}\sum_{i=1}^n \boldsymbol{T}(X^{(i)})\right), \qquad \boldsymbol{\zeta} \in \Xi,\end{aligned}$$

by using the same arguments as in the proof of Theorem 4.26 and that $X^{(1)}, \ldots, X^{(n)}$ are iid. Evidently, $\sum_{i=1}^n \boldsymbol{T}(X^{(i)})/n$ is unbiased for $\pi(\boldsymbol{\zeta})$, $\boldsymbol{\zeta} \in \Xi$, and the assertion follows. □

In particular, Theorem 4.26 and Corollary 4.27 apply to (minimal) regular EFs, in which the mean value parameter can therefore always be estimated efficiently.

Examples: $\mathfrak{poi}(\bullet)$, $\mathfrak{b}(n_0, \bullet)$, $\mathfrak{nb}(r_0, \bullet)$, $\mathcal{E}(\bullet)$

Example 4.28 Let $\mathcal{P}$ be any of the EFs $\mathfrak{poi}(\bullet)$, $\mathfrak{b}(n_0, \bullet)$, $\mathfrak{nb}(r_0, \bullet)$, or $\mathcal{E}(\bullet)$ in Examples 2.37, 2.38, 2.51, and 2.12. Moreover, let $X_1, \ldots, X_n$ be an iid sample from $P_\zeta^* \in \mathcal{P}$. Then, by Corollary 4.27, $\sum_{i=1}^n X_i/n$ is an efficient estimator (and thus a UMVUE) for the mean of P_ζ^*.

4.4 Asymptotic Properties

In the examples of Sect. 4.1, the probability that the ML estimate of $\boldsymbol{\zeta}$ in Ξ^* based on n observations exists is equal to 1 or at least converges to 1 when the sample size tends to infinity. This finding holds true in general for minimal regular EFs. It is a consequence of the following theorem.

Theorem 4.29 *Let $\mathcal{P}$ be an EF with minimal canonical representation (4.1), $\Xi \subset \Xi^*$ be open, and $X^{(1)}, X^{(2)}, \ldots$ be a sequence of iid random variables with distribution $P^*_{\boldsymbol{\zeta}} \in \mathcal{P}$ for some $\boldsymbol{\zeta} \in \Xi$. Then,*

$$\lim_{n\to\infty} \mathbb{P}_{\boldsymbol{\zeta}}\left(\frac{1}{n}\sum_{i=1}^{n} \boldsymbol{T}(X^{(i)}) \in \pi(\Xi)\right) = 1\,,$$

i.e., the probability that the ML estimate of $\boldsymbol{\zeta}$ in Ξ based on realizations $x^{(1)}, \ldots, x^{(n)}$ of $X^{(1)}, \ldots, X^{(n)}$ exists converges to 1 for $n \to \infty$.

Proof Let $\boldsymbol{\zeta} \in \Xi$. By Theorem 2.49, all moments of $\boldsymbol{T}$ with respect to $P^*_{\boldsymbol{\zeta}}$ are finite. The strong law of large numbers together with the definition of π in Theorem 2.56 then yields that

$$\frac{1}{n}\sum_{i=1}^{n} \boldsymbol{T}(X^{(i)}) \overset{n\to\infty}{\longrightarrow} \mathbb{E}_{\boldsymbol{\zeta}}[\boldsymbol{T}(X^{(1)})] = \pi(\boldsymbol{\zeta}) \qquad \mathbb{P}_{\boldsymbol{\zeta}}\text{-a.s.}\,,$$

which implies that $\sum_{i=1}^{n} \boldsymbol{T}(X^{(i)})/n \to \pi(\boldsymbol{\zeta})$ in $\mathbb{P}_{\boldsymbol{\zeta}}$-probability (see, e.g., [55, p. 51]). Moreover, by Theorem 2.56, π^{-1} is continuous, and we conclude that $\pi(\Xi)$ is open as the pre-image $(\pi^{-1})^{-1}(\Xi) = \{\boldsymbol{m} \in \pi(int(\Xi^*)) : \pi^{-1}(\boldsymbol{m}) \in \Xi\}$ of the open set Ξ under π^{-1}. Hence, there exist some $\varepsilon > 0$ and an Euclidean ball $B_\varepsilon(\pi(\boldsymbol{\zeta})) = \{\boldsymbol{\eta} \in \mathbb{R}^k : ||\boldsymbol{\eta} - \pi(\boldsymbol{\zeta})||_2 < \varepsilon\} \subset \pi(\Xi)$. Now, it follows that

$$\begin{aligned}
\mathbb{P}_{\boldsymbol{\zeta}}\left(\frac{1}{n}\sum_{i=1}^{n} \boldsymbol{T}(X^{(i)}) \in \pi(\Xi)\right) &\geq \mathbb{P}_{\boldsymbol{\zeta}}\left(\frac{1}{n}\sum_{i=1}^{n} \boldsymbol{T}(X^{(i)}) \in B_\varepsilon(\pi(\boldsymbol{\zeta}))\right) \\
&= 1 - \mathbb{P}_{\boldsymbol{\zeta}}\left(\left|\left|\frac{1}{n}\sum_{i=1}^{n} \boldsymbol{T}(X^{(i)}) - \pi(\boldsymbol{\zeta})\right|\right|_2 \geq \varepsilon\right) \\
&\overset{n\to\infty}{\longrightarrow} 1\,.
\end{aligned}$$

Finally, since Ξ is open, Lemma 4.2 yields that an ML estimate of $\boldsymbol{\zeta}$ in Ξ based on realizations $x^{(1)}, \ldots, x^{(n)}$ of $X^{(1)}, \ldots, X^{(n)}$ exists (and is then uniquely determined) if and only if the corresponding likelihood equation $\pi(\cdot) = \sum_{i=1}^{n} \boldsymbol{T}(x^{(i)})/n$ has a solution in Ξ. This completes the proof. □

In Sect. 4.3, we have shown that the parameter $\boldsymbol{m} = \pi(\boldsymbol{\zeta})$ of the mean value parametrization can be estimated efficiently in minimal regular EFs. Based on a single random variable $X \sim \tilde{P}_{\boldsymbol{m}} = P^*_{\pi^{-1}(\boldsymbol{m})}$, for example, $\boldsymbol{T}(X)$ was proven to form an efficient estimator for $\boldsymbol{m}$. In contrast, provided that it exists in Ξ^* with probability 1, the MLE $\pi^{-1}(\boldsymbol{T}(X))$ of the natural parameter does not have to be efficient, not even unbiased for $\boldsymbol{\zeta}$ in general. Asymptotically, however, it possesses prominent properties, which are introduced in what follows.

First, the consistency of an estimator, more precisely of a sequence of estimators, is the property that the estimator approaches the true parameter when the sample size increases.

Definition 4.30 Let $\gamma : \Xi \to \mathbb{R}^q$ be a function and $\hat{\gamma}^{(n)} : (\Omega, \mathcal{A}, \mathbb{P}_{\boldsymbol{\zeta}}) \to (\mathbb{R}^q, \mathbb{B}^q)$ be an estimator of γ for every $n \in \mathbb{N}$. Then, the sequence $\hat{\gamma}^{(n)}$, $n \in \mathbb{N}$, is called *(strongly) consistent for* γ if

$$\hat{\gamma}^{(n)} \stackrel{n\to\infty}{\longrightarrow} \gamma(\boldsymbol{\zeta})$$

in $\mathbb{P}_{\boldsymbol{\zeta}}$-probability ($\mathbb{P}_{\boldsymbol{\zeta}}$-a.s.) for every $\boldsymbol{\zeta} \in \Xi$.

In particular, a sequence $\hat{\boldsymbol{\zeta}}^{(n)}$, $n \in \mathbb{N}$, of estimators is called *(strongly) consistent for* $\boldsymbol{\zeta}$ if

$$\hat{\boldsymbol{\zeta}}^{(n)} \stackrel{n\to\infty}{\longrightarrow} \boldsymbol{\zeta}$$

in $\mathbb{P}_{\boldsymbol{\zeta}}$-probability ($\mathbb{P}_{\boldsymbol{\zeta}}$-a.s.) for every $\boldsymbol{\zeta} \in \Xi$.

Note that strong consistency implies consistency by definition.

Theorem 4.31 *Let $\mathcal{P}$ be a regular EF with minimal canonical representation (4.1) and $X^{(1)}, X^{(2)}, \ldots$ be a sequence of iid random variables with distribution $P^*_{\boldsymbol{\zeta}} \in \mathcal{P}$. Moreover, let the MLE $\hat{\boldsymbol{\zeta}}^{(n)}$ of $\boldsymbol{\zeta}$ in Ξ^* based on $X^{(1)}, \ldots, X^{(n)}$ exist for every $n \in \mathbb{N}$. Then, the sequence $\hat{\boldsymbol{\zeta}}^{(n)}$, $n \in \mathbb{N}$, is strongly consistent for $\boldsymbol{\zeta}$.*

Proof Let $\boldsymbol{\zeta} \in \Xi^*$. As in the proof of Theorem 4.29, we have

$$\frac{1}{n}\sum_{i=1}^{n} \boldsymbol{T}(X^{(i)}) \longrightarrow \pi(\boldsymbol{\zeta}) \qquad \mathbb{P}_{\boldsymbol{\zeta}}\text{-a.s.}.$$

Since π^{-1} is continuous by Theorem 2.56, we obtain from formula (4.3) that

$$\hat{\boldsymbol{\zeta}}^{(n)} = \pi^{-1}\left(\frac{1}{n}\sum_{i=1}^{n} \boldsymbol{T}(X^{(i)})\right) \overset{n\to\infty}{\longrightarrow} \pi^{-1}(\pi(\boldsymbol{\zeta})) = \boldsymbol{\zeta} \qquad \mathbb{P}_{\boldsymbol{\zeta}}\text{-a.s.}.$$

□

Another main concept for sequences of estimators is asymptotic efficiency, which is motivated by Definition 4.21.

Definition 4.32 Let $\Xi \subset \Xi^*$ be open, $\gamma : \Xi \to \mathbb{R}^q$ be a differentiable function with Jacobian matrix $\mathbf{D}_\gamma(\boldsymbol{\zeta}) \in \mathbb{R}^{q\times k}$ of rank q at every $\boldsymbol{\zeta} \in \Xi$, and $\hat{\gamma}^{(n)} : (\Omega, \mathcal{A}, \mathbb{P}_{\boldsymbol{\zeta}}) \to (\mathbb{R}^q, \mathbb{B}^q)$ be an estimator of γ for every $n \in \mathbb{N}$. Then, the sequence $\hat{\gamma}^{(n)}$, $n \in \mathbb{N}$, is called *asymptotically efficient for* γ if

$$\sqrt{n}\,(\hat{\gamma}^{(n)} - \gamma(\boldsymbol{\zeta})) \overset{d}{\longrightarrow} N_q(\mathbf{0}, \mathbf{D}_\gamma(\boldsymbol{\zeta})[\mathbf{I}(\boldsymbol{\zeta})]^{-1}\mathbf{D}_\gamma(\boldsymbol{\zeta})^t) \qquad \text{for } \boldsymbol{\zeta} \in \Xi\,,$$

i.e., $\sqrt{n}(\hat{\gamma}^{(n)} - \gamma(\boldsymbol{\zeta}))$ is asymptotically multivariate normal distributed with mean vector $\mathbf{0}$ and covariance matrix $\mathbf{D}_\gamma(\boldsymbol{\zeta})[\mathbf{I}(\boldsymbol{\zeta})]^{-1}\mathbf{D}_\gamma(\boldsymbol{\zeta})^t$.

In particular, a sequence $\hat{\boldsymbol{\zeta}}^{(n)}$, $n \in \mathbb{N}$, of estimators is called *asymptotically efficient for* $\boldsymbol{\zeta}$ if

$$\sqrt{n}\,(\hat{\boldsymbol{\zeta}}^{(n)} - \boldsymbol{\zeta}) \overset{d}{\longrightarrow} N_k(\mathbf{0}, [\mathbf{I}(\boldsymbol{\zeta})]^{-1}) \qquad \text{for } \boldsymbol{\zeta} \in \Xi\,.$$

Here, $\mathbf{I}(\boldsymbol{\zeta})$ denotes the Fisher information matrix of $\mathcal{P}$ at $\boldsymbol{\zeta}$, which is assumed to be regular for all $\boldsymbol{\zeta} \in \Xi$.

Remark 4.33 We shall address some motivational aspects for Definition 4.32 (see also [39, pp. 437–443]). Suppose that $\hat{\boldsymbol{\zeta}}^{(n)}$, $n \in \mathbb{N}$, is asymptotically efficient for $\boldsymbol{\zeta}$ according to Definition 4.32. If we further assume that the covariance matrix of $\sqrt{n}(\hat{\boldsymbol{\zeta}}^{(n)} - \boldsymbol{\zeta})$ converges to that of the asymptotic distribution for $n \to \infty$, this yields for sufficiently large n that

$$[\mathbf{I}(\boldsymbol{\zeta})]^{-1} \approx \mathbb{C}\mathrm{ov}_{\boldsymbol{\zeta}}\left(\sqrt{n}(\hat{\boldsymbol{\zeta}}^{(n)} - \boldsymbol{\zeta})\right) = n\,\mathbb{C}\mathrm{ov}_{\boldsymbol{\zeta}}\left(\hat{\boldsymbol{\zeta}}^{(n)}\right), \qquad \boldsymbol{\zeta} \in \Xi\,.$$

That is, the covariance matrix of $\hat{\boldsymbol{\zeta}}^{(n)}$ approximately attains the lower bound $[\mathbf{I}(\boldsymbol{\zeta})]^{-1}/n$ of the Cramér-Rao inequality for $\mathcal{P}^{(n)}$ related to an iid sample of size n (see Sect. 4.3). Note, however, that $\hat{\boldsymbol{\zeta}}^{(n)}$ is not necessarily unbiased for $\boldsymbol{\zeta}$.

In a minimal regular EF, it can moreover be shown that for every sequence $\tilde{\boldsymbol{\zeta}}^{(n)}$, $n \in \mathbb{N}$, of estimators for $\boldsymbol{\zeta}$ with

$$\sqrt{n}\,(\tilde{\boldsymbol{\zeta}}^{(n)} - \boldsymbol{\zeta}) \xrightarrow{d} \mathcal{N}_k(\mathbf{0}, \boldsymbol{\Sigma}(\boldsymbol{\zeta})) \qquad \text{for every } \boldsymbol{\zeta} \in \Xi^*,$$

we necessarily have

$$\boldsymbol{\Sigma}(\boldsymbol{\zeta}) \geq [\mathbf{I}(\boldsymbol{\zeta})]^{-1} \qquad \lambda_{\Xi^*}\text{-a.e.}$$

in the sense of the Löwner order (see [39, pp. 437–443] and the references cited therein). If $\boldsymbol{\Sigma}$ and $\mathbf{I}^{-1}$ are continuous on Ξ^*, then the inequality holds even everywhere on Ξ^*. Hence, an asymptotically efficient sequence of estimators has minimum asymptotic covariance matrix within a certain class of (sequences of) estimators.

Note that asymptotic efficiency implies consistency. This can be seen by rewriting

$$\hat{\boldsymbol{\zeta}}^{(n)} - \boldsymbol{\zeta} = \frac{1}{\sqrt{n}}\sqrt{n}(\hat{\boldsymbol{\zeta}}^{(n)} - \boldsymbol{\zeta}),$$

which converges to $\mathbf{0}$ in distribution by applying the multivariate Slutsky theorem (see, e.g., [53, p. 130]). Since the limit is a constant, this convergence holds true even in $\mathbb{P}_{\boldsymbol{\zeta}}$-probability (see, for instance, [55, p. 51]).

Theorem 4.34 *Under the assumptions of Theorem 4.31, the sequence $\hat{\boldsymbol{\zeta}}^{(n)}$, $n \in \mathbb{N}$, is asymptotically efficient for $\boldsymbol{\zeta}$.*

Proof Let $\boldsymbol{\zeta} \in \Xi^*$. First, recall that by Theorems 2.56 and 3.29, it holds that

$$\mathbb{E}_{\boldsymbol{\zeta}}[\boldsymbol{T}(X^{(1)})] = \boldsymbol{\pi}(\boldsymbol{\zeta}), \qquad \mathbb{C}\mathrm{ov}_{\boldsymbol{\zeta}}(\boldsymbol{T}(X^{(1)})) = \mathbf{I}(\boldsymbol{\zeta}).$$

The multivariate central limit theorem (see, e.g., [55, Section 1.5]) then yields that

$$\sqrt{n}\left(\frac{1}{n}\sum_{i=1}^{n}\boldsymbol{T}(X^{(i)}) - \boldsymbol{\pi}(\boldsymbol{\zeta})\right) \xrightarrow{d} \boldsymbol{N} \tag{4.10}$$

for a random vector $\boldsymbol{N} \sim \mathcal{N}_k(\mathbf{0}, \mathbf{I}(\boldsymbol{\zeta}))$.

Now, to ease notation, let $\boldsymbol{\rho} = (\rho_1, \ldots, \rho_k)$ denote the inverse function of $\boldsymbol{\pi}$, i.e., we have $\boldsymbol{\rho} = \boldsymbol{\pi}^{-1}$. Then, formula (4.3) along with the mean value theorem for real-valued functions of several variables (e.g., in [52, p. 174]) applied to every of the mappings ρ_j, $1 \le j \le k$, yields

$$\sqrt{n}\,(\hat{\boldsymbol{\zeta}}^{(n)} - \boldsymbol{\zeta}) = \sqrt{n}\left(\rho\left(\frac{1}{n}\sum_{i=1}^{n} \boldsymbol{T}(X^{(i)})\right) - \rho(\pi(\boldsymbol{\zeta}))\right)$$

$$= \mathbf{G}_n \sqrt{n}\left(\frac{1}{n}\sum_{i=1}^{n} \boldsymbol{T}(X^{(i)}) - \pi(\boldsymbol{\zeta})\right),$$

where $\mathbf{G}_n$ is a random matrix with rows

$$[\nabla\rho_j(\boldsymbol{V}_j^{(n)})]^t, \qquad 1 \le j \le k,$$

and the random vectors $\boldsymbol{V}_1^{(n)}, \ldots, \boldsymbol{V}_k^{(n)}$ are convex combinations of $\sum_{i=1}^{n} \boldsymbol{T}(X^{(i)})/n$ and $\pi(\boldsymbol{\zeta})$ for $n \in \mathbb{N}$. For $n \to \infty$, the strong law of large numbers ensures that $\sum_{i=1}^{n} \boldsymbol{T}(X^{(i)})/n \to \pi(\boldsymbol{\zeta})\mathbb{P}_{\boldsymbol{\zeta}}$-a.s. and with it $\boldsymbol{V}_j^{(n)} \to \pi(\boldsymbol{\zeta})\mathbb{P}_{\boldsymbol{\zeta}}$-a.s. for $1 \le j \le k$. From Corollary 2.56 and Theorem 3.29, we conclude

$$\mathbf{G}_n \stackrel{n\to\infty}{\longrightarrow} \mathbf{D}_\rho(\pi(\boldsymbol{\zeta})) = [\mathbf{D}_\pi(\boldsymbol{\zeta})]^{-1} = [\mathbf{I}(\boldsymbol{\zeta})]^{-1} \qquad \mathbb{P}_{\boldsymbol{\zeta}}\text{-a.s.}.$$

By the multivariate Slutsky theorem (see, e.g., [53, p. 130]), it finally follows that

$$\sqrt{n}\,(\hat{\boldsymbol{\zeta}}^{(n)} - \boldsymbol{\zeta}) \stackrel{d}{\longrightarrow} [\mathbf{I}(\boldsymbol{\zeta})]^{-1}\boldsymbol{N},$$

and, since $[\mathbf{I}(\boldsymbol{\zeta})]^{-1}\boldsymbol{N} \sim \mathcal{N}_k(\mathbf{0}, [\mathbf{I}(\boldsymbol{\zeta})]^{-1})$, the proof is completed. □

Note that if $\mathcal{P}$ is not assumed to be regular, Theorems 4.31 and 4.34 remain valid when replacing Ξ^* by some open set $\Xi \subset \Xi^*$.

Remark 4.35 The assumption in Theorems 4.31 and 4.34 saying that the MLE $\hat{\boldsymbol{\zeta}}^{(n)}$ of $\boldsymbol{\zeta}$ in Ξ^* based on $X^{(1)}, \ldots, X^{(n)}$ exists for $n \in \mathbb{N}$ may be dropped in a certain sense. Evidently, we may weaken the assumption from all $n \in \mathbb{N}$ to eventually all $n \in \mathbb{N}$, i.e., for all $n \ge n_0$ for some $n_0 \in \mathbb{N}$, without affecting the findings. If even the latter property is not met, we may proceed as follows to obtain a strongly consistent and asymptotically efficient estimator for $\boldsymbol{\zeta}$.

Let $\boldsymbol{t} \in \pi(\Xi^*)$ be arbitrary. Moreover, for $n \in \mathbb{N}$, we introduce the set

$$A_n = \left\{\frac{1}{n}\sum_{i=1}^{n} \boldsymbol{T}(X^{(i)}) \in \pi(\Xi^*)\right\} \in \mathcal{A}$$

and the estimator

$$\tilde{\boldsymbol{\zeta}}^{(n)} = \pi^{-1}(\boldsymbol{W}_n) \qquad \text{with} \qquad \boldsymbol{W}_n = \left(\frac{1}{n}\sum_{i=1}^{n} \boldsymbol{T}(X^{(i)})\right)\mathbb{1}_{A_n} + \boldsymbol{t}\,\mathbb{1}_{A_n^c}.$$

Now, for $\boldsymbol{\zeta} \in \Xi^*$, we have that $\sum_{i=1}^n \boldsymbol{T}(X^{(i)})/n \to \pi(\boldsymbol{\zeta})\mathbb{P}_{\boldsymbol{\zeta}}$-a.s. for $n \to \infty$ by the strong law of large numbers. Since $\pi(\Xi^*) = int(M)$ is open, this implies that $\mathbb{1}_{A_n} \to 1\mathbb{P}_{\boldsymbol{\zeta}}$-a.s. and $\mathbb{1}_{A_n^c} \to 0\mathbb{P}_{\boldsymbol{\zeta}}$-a.s. for $n \to \infty$. Hence,

$$\boldsymbol{W}_n \overset{n\to\infty}{\longrightarrow} \pi(\boldsymbol{\zeta}) \qquad \mathbb{P}_{\boldsymbol{\zeta}}\text{-a.s.}, \tag{4.11}$$

and, since π^{-1} is continuous by Theorem 2.56, it follows that $\tilde{\boldsymbol{\zeta}}^{(n)} \to \boldsymbol{\zeta}\mathbb{P}_{\boldsymbol{\zeta}}$-a.s. for $n \to \infty$, i.e., the sequence $\tilde{\boldsymbol{\zeta}}^{(n)}$, $n \in \mathbb{N}$, is strongly consistent for $\boldsymbol{\zeta}$.

To establish that the sequence $\tilde{\boldsymbol{\zeta}}^{(n)}$, $n \in \mathbb{N}$, is also asymptotically efficient for $\boldsymbol{\zeta}$, note first that for $n \in \mathbb{N}$

$$\boldsymbol{W}_n = \frac{1}{n}\sum_{i=1}^n \boldsymbol{T}(X^{(i)}) + \left(\boldsymbol{t} - \frac{1}{n}\sum_{i=1}^n \boldsymbol{T}(X^{(i)})\right)\mathbb{1}_{A_n^c}$$

and thus

$$\sqrt{n}(\boldsymbol{W}_n - \pi(\boldsymbol{\zeta})) = \sqrt{n}\left(\frac{1}{n}\sum_{i=1}^n \boldsymbol{T}(X^{(i)}) - \pi(\boldsymbol{\zeta})\right) + \sqrt{n}\left(\boldsymbol{t} - \frac{1}{n}\sum_{i=1}^n \boldsymbol{T}(X^{(i)})\right)\mathbb{1}_{A_n^c}.$$

Since $\mathbb{1}_{A_n^c} \to 0\mathbb{P}_{\boldsymbol{\zeta}}$-a.s. for $n \to \infty$, there exists $\mathbb{P}_{\boldsymbol{\zeta}}$-a.s. an index $m \in \mathbb{N}$ with $\mathbb{1}_{A_n^c} = 0$ for all $n \geq m$. Hence,

$$\sqrt{n}\left(\boldsymbol{t} - \frac{1}{n}\sum_{i=1}^n \boldsymbol{T}(X^{(i)})\right)\mathbb{1}_{A_n^c} \overset{n\to\infty}{\longrightarrow} \boldsymbol{0} \qquad \mathbb{P}_{\boldsymbol{\zeta}}\text{-a.s.}.$$

Formula (4.10) together with the multivariate Slutsky theorem then yields that

$$\sqrt{n}\,(\boldsymbol{W}_n - \pi(\boldsymbol{\zeta})) \overset{d}{\longrightarrow} \mathcal{N}_k(\boldsymbol{0}, \mathbf{I}(\boldsymbol{\zeta})). \tag{4.12}$$

As in the proof of Theorem 4.34, it now follows with $\rho = \pi^{-1}$ that

$$\begin{aligned}\sqrt{n}\,(\tilde{\boldsymbol{\zeta}}^{(n)} - \boldsymbol{\zeta}) &= \sqrt{n}\,(\rho(\boldsymbol{W}_n) - \rho(\pi(\boldsymbol{\zeta}))) \\ &= \tilde{\mathbf{G}}_n \sqrt{n}\,(\boldsymbol{W}_n - \pi(\boldsymbol{\zeta})),\end{aligned}$$

where $\tilde{\mathbf{G}}_n$ is a random matrix with rows

$$[\nabla\rho_j(\tilde{\boldsymbol{V}}_j^{(n)})]^t, \qquad 1 \leq j \leq k,$$

and the random vectors $\tilde{\boldsymbol{V}}_1^{(n)}, \ldots, \tilde{\boldsymbol{V}}_k^{(n)}$ are convex combinations of $\boldsymbol{W}_n$ and $\pi(\boldsymbol{\zeta})$ for $n \in \mathbb{N}$. From formula (4.11), we obtain for $n \to \infty$ that $\tilde{\boldsymbol{V}}_j^{(n)} \to \pi(\boldsymbol{\zeta})\mathbb{P}_{\boldsymbol{\zeta}}$-a.s.

for $1 \le j \le k$ and thus $\tilde{\mathbf{G}}_n \to [\mathbf{I}(\boldsymbol{\zeta})]^{-1}\mathbb{P}_{\boldsymbol{\zeta}}$-a.s. as in the proof of Theorem 4.34. The latter finding together with formula (4.12) then yields that

$$\sqrt{n}\,(\tilde{\boldsymbol{\zeta}}^{(n)} - \boldsymbol{\zeta}) \xrightarrow{d} \mathcal{N}_k(\mathbf{0}, [\mathbf{I}(\boldsymbol{\zeta})]^{-1})$$

by using the multivariate Slutsky theorem, again. Thus, asymptotic efficiency of $\tilde{\boldsymbol{\zeta}}^{(n)}$, $n \in \mathbb{N}$, is shown.

Asymptotic properties for curved EFs are stated in the following remark.

Remark 4.36 Let $\mathcal{P}_{\mathbf{Z}} \subset \mathcal{P}$ with $\mathbf{Z} : \Theta \to \Xi^*$ be a curved EF as introduced in Remark 4.14, where we assume that $\mathbf{Z}(\Theta) \subset int(\Xi^*)$ and that $\mathbf{Z}(\Theta)$ is relatively closed in Ξ^*. Moreover, suppose that the MLE $\hat{\vartheta}_n$ of ϑ in $\Theta \subset \mathbb{R}^m$ based on a sample of size n uniquely exists for eventually all $n \in \mathbb{N}$. Then the sequence $\hat{\vartheta}_n$, $n \in \mathbb{N}$, is strongly consistent provided that $\mathbf{Z}$ has a continuous inverse $\mathbf{Z}^{-1}$: $\mathbf{Z}(\Theta) \to \Theta$. If, in addition, Θ is open and $\mathbf{Z}$ is continuously differentiable with Jacobian matrix $\mathbf{D}_{\mathbf{Z}}(\vartheta)$ of full rank m at every $\vartheta \in \Theta$, then $\sqrt{n}(\hat{\vartheta}_n - \vartheta)$ converges in distribution to $\mathcal{N}_m(\mathbf{0}, [\mathbf{D}_{\mathbf{Z}}(\vartheta)^t \mathbf{I}(\mathbf{Z}(\vartheta))\mathbf{D}_{\mathbf{Z}}(\vartheta)]^{-1})$. Here, $\mathbf{I}(\mathbf{Z}(\vartheta))$ denotes the Fisher information matrix of $\mathcal{P}$ at $\mathbf{Z}(\vartheta)$. For a detailed discussion along with proofs of the above results, see, e.g., [14].

Having proposed strongly consistent and asymptotically efficient sequences of estimators for the natural parameter $\boldsymbol{\zeta}$ of the EF, we finally state sufficient conditions under which these properties transfer to a sequence of estimators for $\gamma(\boldsymbol{\zeta})$.

Lemma 4.37 *Let $\mathcal{P}$ be an EF with minimal canonical representation (4.1), $\Xi \subset \Xi^*$ be open, and $\gamma : \Xi \to \mathbb{R}^q$ be a mapping. Moreover, let $\tilde{\boldsymbol{\zeta}}^{(n)}$, $n \in \mathbb{N}$, be a sequence of estimators for $\boldsymbol{\zeta}$. Then, the following assertions hold true:*

(a) If $\tilde{\boldsymbol{\zeta}}^{(n)}$, $n \in \mathbb{N}$, is strongly consistent for $\boldsymbol{\zeta}$ and γ is continuous, then the sequence $\gamma(\tilde{\boldsymbol{\zeta}}^{(n)})$, $n \in \mathbb{N}$, is strongly consistent for γ.

(b) If $\tilde{\boldsymbol{\zeta}}^{(n)}$, $n \in \mathbb{N}$, is asymptotically efficient for $\boldsymbol{\zeta}$ and γ is continuously differentiable with Jacobian matrix $\mathbf{D}_\gamma(\boldsymbol{\zeta}) \in \mathbb{R}^{q\times k}$ of rank q at every $\boldsymbol{\zeta} \in \Xi$, then the sequence $\gamma(\tilde{\boldsymbol{\zeta}}^{(n)})$, $n \in \mathbb{N}$, is asymptotically efficient for γ.

Proof Assertion (a) is clear, since a.s.-convergence is preserved under continuous mappings. To show assertion (b), let γ be continuously differentiable and $\boldsymbol{\zeta} \in \Xi$. Then, applying the mean value theorem for real-valued functions of several variables (e.g., in [52, p. 174]) to γ_j for $1 \le j \le q$ gives

$$\sqrt{n}\,(\gamma(\tilde{\boldsymbol{\zeta}}^{(n)}) - \gamma(\boldsymbol{\zeta})) = \check{\mathbf{G}}_n \sqrt{n}\left(\tilde{\boldsymbol{\zeta}}^{(n)} - \boldsymbol{\zeta}\right),$$

where $\check{\mathbf{G}}_n$ is a random matrix with rows

$$[\nabla\gamma_j(\check{\mathbf{V}}_j^{(n)})]^t, \qquad 1 \le j \le q,$$

and the random vectors $\check{V}_1^{(n)}, \ldots, \check{V}_q^{(n)}$ are convex combinations of $\tilde{\boldsymbol{\xi}}^{(n)}$ and $\boldsymbol{\zeta}$ for $n \in \mathbb{N}$. Since $\tilde{\boldsymbol{\xi}}^{(n)}$, $n \in \mathbb{N}$, is assumed to be asymptotically efficient, it is also consistent for $\boldsymbol{\zeta}$, i.e., we have $\tilde{\boldsymbol{\xi}}^{(n)} \to \boldsymbol{\zeta}$ in $\mathbb{P}_{\boldsymbol{\zeta}}$-probability for $n \to \infty$. Consequently, for $1 \leq j \leq q$, we also have $\check{V}_j^{(n)} \to \boldsymbol{\zeta}$ in $\mathbb{P}_{\boldsymbol{\zeta}}$-probability for $n \to \infty$. Moreover, for $1 \leq j \leq q$, $\nabla\gamma_j$ is continuous by assumption, which implies that

$$\check{\mathbf{G}}_n \overset{n\to\infty}{\longrightarrow} \mathbf{D}_\gamma(\boldsymbol{\zeta}) \qquad \text{in } \mathbb{P}_{\boldsymbol{\zeta}}\text{-probability}$$

by using that convergence in probability is preserved under continuous mappings (see, e.g., [55, p. 59]). Since $\tilde{\boldsymbol{\xi}}^{(n)}$, $n \in \mathbb{N}$, is asymptotically efficient for $\boldsymbol{\zeta}$, applying the multivariate Slutsky theorem finally gives

$$\sqrt{n}\,(\gamma(\tilde{\boldsymbol{\xi}}^{(n)}) - \gamma(\boldsymbol{\zeta})) \overset{d}{\longrightarrow} \mathcal{N}_q(\mathbf{0}, \mathbf{D}_\gamma(\boldsymbol{\zeta})[\mathbf{I}(\boldsymbol{\zeta})]^{-1}\mathbf{D}_\gamma(\boldsymbol{\zeta})^t)\,,$$

i.e., $\gamma(\tilde{\boldsymbol{\xi}}^{(n)})$, $n \in \mathbb{N}$, is asymptotically efficient for γ. □

Chapter 5
Hypotheses Testing

As a basic concept of statistical inference, a statistical test allows for a data-based decision between two contrary hypotheses about some population, where two error probabilities with opposing trends are fundamental.

In a one-parameter EF, uniformly most powerful tests are easily found for particular, but important hypotheses. Moreover, uniformly most powerful unbiased tests can be established in other cases and in multiparameter EFs as well via conditioning, which reduces the problem to the one-parameter case. Finally, statistical tests for several parameters simultaneously are considered with a focus on likelihood-ratio tests.

For a rigorous introduction in hypotheses testing, we refer to the rich textbook literature on Mathematical Statistics. In order to become familiar with the topic, a basic knowledge of statistical testing with some applications is helpful.

5.1 One-Sided Test Problems

Definition 5.1 Let $\mathcal{P} = \{P^*_\zeta : \zeta \in \Xi\}$ be a family of distributions on the measurable space $(\mathcal{X}, \mathcal{B})$.

(a) Every $(\mathcal{B} - \mathbb{B}^1)$-measurable mapping $\varphi : \mathcal{X} \to [0, 1]$ is called a *(statistical) test*, and the function β_φ defined by

(continued)

S. Bedbur, U. Kamps, *Multivariate Exponential Families: A Concise Guide to Statistical Inference*, SpringerBriefs in Statistics,
https://doi.org/10.1007/978-3-030-81900-2_5

Definition 5.1 (continued)

$$\beta_\varphi(\boldsymbol{\zeta}) = E_{\boldsymbol{\zeta}}[\varphi] = \int \varphi \, dP^*_{\boldsymbol{\zeta}}\,, \qquad \boldsymbol{\zeta} \in \Xi\,,$$

is its *power function.*

If φ only takes on the values 0 and 1, then it is called *non-randomized.*

(b) For non-empty, disjoint subsets Ξ_0 and Ξ_1 of Ξ, the test problem with *null hypothesis* $H_0 : \boldsymbol{\zeta} \in \Xi_0$ and *alternative hypothesis* $H_1 : \boldsymbol{\zeta} \in \Xi_1$ is denoted by

$$H_0 : \boldsymbol{\zeta} \in \Xi_0 \qquad \leftrightarrow \qquad H_1 : \boldsymbol{\zeta} \in \Xi_1\,. \tag{5.1}$$

A test φ is then said to have *(significance) level* $\alpha \in (0, 1)$ for test problem (5.1) if

$$\beta_\varphi(\boldsymbol{\zeta}) \leq \alpha \qquad \text{for all } \boldsymbol{\zeta} \in \Xi_0\,,$$

and a test φ with level $\alpha \in (0, 1)$ for test problem (5.1) is called *unbiased* if

$$\beta_\varphi(\boldsymbol{\zeta}) \geq \alpha \qquad \text{for all } \boldsymbol{\zeta} \in \Xi_1\,.$$

Roughly speaking, $\varphi(x)$ is interpreted as the probability to decide for the alternative hypothesis H_1 if $x \in \mathcal{X}$ has been observed. $\varphi(x) = 0$ therefore corresponds to a decision for H_0, whereas $\varphi(x) = 1$ yields a decision for H_1. If there exists some $x \in \mathcal{X}$ for which $\varphi(x) \in (0, 1)$, then φ is called a *randomized test*, in the case of which the decision is indeed random and has to be implemented by some additional rule; one may think of flipping a fair coin in case of $\varphi(x) = 1/2$ as a simple example. Allowing for randomization of the test decision is useful in the derivation of optimal tests; in practice, however, they do not play an important role and are usually avoided by adjusting the level of the test.

For $\boldsymbol{\zeta} \in \Xi_0$, $\beta_\varphi(\boldsymbol{\zeta})$ is called the *error probability of the first kind* of φ at $\boldsymbol{\zeta}$; for a non-randomized test, it is the probability of deciding in favor of H_1 and the true parameter is in Ξ_0. Accordingly, for $\boldsymbol{\zeta} \in \Xi_1$, $1-\beta_\varphi(\boldsymbol{\zeta})$ is called the *error probability of the second kind* of φ at $\boldsymbol{\zeta}$; for a non-randomized test, it is the probability of deciding in favor of H_0 and the true parameter is in Ξ_1. In the latter case, $\beta_\varphi(\boldsymbol{\zeta})$ is also said to be the *power* of φ at $\boldsymbol{\zeta}$. Usually, it is not possible to simultaneously minimize the error probabilities of the first and second kind. The derivation of optimal tests is therefore based on a non-symmetric procedure. One minimizes the error probability of the second kind—and thus maximizes power—in a restricted family of tests, for example, among all tests with the same level.

Definition 5.2 Let Φ be a set of statistical tests. A test $\varphi \in \Phi$ is called *uniformly most powerful (UMP) in Φ for test problem (5.1)* if

$$\beta_{\varphi}(\boldsymbol{\zeta}) = \sup_{\psi \in \Phi} \beta_{\psi}(\boldsymbol{\zeta}) \qquad \text{for all } \boldsymbol{\zeta} \in \Xi_1 .$$

For the particular case

$$\Phi = \{\psi : \psi \text{ is a test with level } \alpha \text{ for test problem (5.1)}\} ,$$

φ is called a *UMP (uniformly most powerful) level-α test*, and for

$$\Phi = \{\psi : \psi \text{ is an unbiased test with level } \alpha \text{ for test problem (5.1)}\} ,$$

φ is called a *UMPU (uniformly most powerful unbiased) level-α test for test problem (5.1).*

Note that a UMP level-α test is necessarily unbiased, since its power is not smaller than that of the constant level-α test $\psi \equiv \alpha$ at every $\boldsymbol{\zeta} \in \Xi_1$. As a consequence, every UMP level-α test is also a UMPU level-α test.

For one- and multiparameter regular EFs, UMP or UMPU level-α tests can be provided for various test problems concerning a single parameter. These optimal tests are readily deduced from the (generalized) Neyman-Pearson lemma, which is presented in what follows. For the proof, see, e.g., [63, Section 2.4.].

Lemma 5.3 *Let μ be a σ-finite measure and $f_0, f_1, \ldots, f_n$ be real-valued, μ-integrable functions on the measurable space $(\mathcal{X}, \mathcal{B})$ for some $n \in \mathbb{N}$. Moreover, assume that $(\alpha_0, \alpha_1, \ldots, \alpha_{n-1}) \in int(Q)$ with*

$$Q = \left\{(q_0, q_1, \ldots, q_{n-1}) \in \mathbb{R}^n : \textit{there exists a test } \psi \textit{ with} \right.$$
$$\left. \int \psi f_i \, d\mu = q_i \ \textit{ for all } \ i = 0, 1, \ldots, n-1 \right\}.$$

Then, the following properties hold true:

(a) A test φ maximizes $\int \psi f_n \, d\mu$ among all tests ψ in

$$\Phi = \{\psi : \psi \textit{ is test with} \int \psi f_i \, d\mu = \alpha_i \ , \ i = 0, 1, \ldots, n-1\}$$

if and only if there exist constants $k_0, k_1, \ldots, k_{n-1} \in \mathbb{R}$ *with*

$$\varphi(x) = \begin{cases} 1, & f_n(x) > \sum_{i=0}^{n-1} k_i f_i(x), \\ 0, & f_n(x) < \sum_{i=0}^{n-1} k_i f_i(x), \end{cases} \qquad \mu\text{-a.e.}. \tag{5.2}$$

(b) There exists a maximizing test φ *according to (a).*

(c) If $\alpha_i = \alpha \int f_i d\mu$ *for* $i = 0, 1, \ldots, n-1$ *and some* $\alpha \in (0, 1)$, *then a test* φ *satisfying formula (5.2) with* $k_0, k_1, \ldots, k_{n-1} \geq 0$ *maximizes* $\int \psi f_n \, d\mu$ *even among all tests* ψ *in*

$$\tilde{\Phi} = \{\psi : \psi \text{ is test with } \int \psi f_i \, d\mu \leq \alpha_i \,, \; i = 0, 1, \ldots, n-1\}.$$

First, we focus on optimal tests in one-parameter EFs, where UMP level-α tests for *one-sided* test problems are derived by applying Lemma 5.3. In what follows, as commonly used, a hypothesis $\zeta \in (-\infty, \zeta_0] \cap \Xi^*$, say, is denoted by $\zeta \leq \zeta_0$, for short.

Theorem 5.4 *Let* $\mathcal{P} = \{P_\zeta^* = f_\zeta^* \mu : \zeta \in \Xi^*\}$ *be a regular EF with* μ*-densities*

$$f_\zeta^*(x) = C^*(\zeta) \, e^{\zeta T(x)} \, h(x) \,, \qquad x \in \mathcal{X},$$

for $\zeta \in \Xi^* \subset \mathbb{R}$. *Moreover, let* $\zeta_0 \in \Xi^*$ *and* $\alpha \in (0, 1)$. *Then, we have:*

(a) For the one-sided test problem

$$H_0 : \zeta \leq \zeta_0 \qquad \leftrightarrow \qquad H_1 : \zeta > \zeta_0 \,, \tag{5.3}$$

a UMP level-α *test is given by*

$$\varphi(x) = \mathbb{1}_{(c,\infty)}(T(x)) + \gamma \, \mathbb{1}_{\{c\}}(T(x)) \,, \qquad x \in \mathcal{X}.$$

(b) For the one-sided test problem

$$H_0 : \zeta \geq \zeta_0 \qquad \leftrightarrow \qquad H_1 : \zeta < \zeta_0 \,,$$

a UMP level-α *test is given by*

$$\varphi(x) = \mathbb{1}_{(-\infty,c)}(T(x)) + \gamma \, \mathbb{1}_{\{c\}}(T(x)) \,, \qquad x \in \mathcal{X}.$$

In (a) and (b), respectively, the constants $c \in \mathbb{R}$ *and* $\gamma \in [0, 1]$ *are each determined by the equation*

$$E_{\zeta_0}[\varphi] = \alpha \,.$$

Proof (a) Let φ be as stated. Without loss of generality, we may assume that $h(x) > 0$ for all $x \in \mathcal{X}$, since $P^*_\zeta(h = 0) = 0$ for $\zeta \in \Xi^*$. We first show that, for every fixed $\zeta_1 \in \Xi^*$ with $\zeta_1 > \zeta_0$, φ is a UMP level-α test for the test problem

$$\tilde{H}_0 : \zeta = \zeta_0 \quad \leftrightarrow \quad \tilde{H}_1 : \zeta = \zeta_1 \tag{5.4}$$

with two *simple* hypotheses ($\Xi_0 = \{\zeta_0\}$ and $\Xi_1 = \{\zeta_1\}$ are singletons).

Obviously, the likelihood ratio

$$\frac{f^*_{\zeta_1}(x)}{f^*_{\zeta_0}(x)} = \frac{C^*(\zeta_1)}{C^*(\zeta_0)} e^{(\zeta_1 - \zeta_0)\, T(x)}$$

is a strictly increasing function in $T(x)$. φ can therefore equivalently be represented as

$$\varphi(x) = \begin{cases} 1, & f^*_{\zeta_1}(x) > k_0\, f^*_{\zeta_0}(x), \\ \gamma, & f^*_{\zeta_1}(x) = k_0\, f^*_{\zeta_0}(x), \\ 0, & f^*_{\zeta_1}(x) < k_0\, f^*_{\zeta_0}(x), \end{cases}$$

for some constant $k_0 \in \mathbb{R}$ such that $E_{\zeta_0}[\varphi] = \alpha$. Necessarily, it holds that $k_0 \geq 0$. Applying Lemma 5.3(c) with $n = 1$, $f_i = f^*_{\zeta_i}$, $i = 0, 1$, and $\alpha_0 = \alpha$ ($Q = [0, 1]$), φ then maximizes

$$\beta_\psi(\zeta_1) = E_{\zeta_1}[\psi] = \int \psi\, f^*_{\zeta_1}\, d\mu$$

among all tests ψ with

$$\beta_\psi(\zeta_0) = E_{\zeta_0}[\psi] = \int \psi\, f^*_{\zeta_0}\, d\mu \leq \alpha\,.$$

By Definitions 5.1 and 5.2, this means that φ is a UMP level-α test for test problem (5.4).

Moreover, since φ does not depend on the special value of $\zeta_1 > \zeta_0$, it is clear from Definition 5.2 that φ is even a UMP level-α test for the test problem

$$\tilde{H}_0 : \zeta = \zeta_0 \quad \leftrightarrow \quad H_1 : \zeta > \zeta_0\,. \tag{5.5}$$

Now, note that every level-α test for test problem (5.3) is a level-α test for test problem (5.5), too. Hence, what is left to verify for φ to be a UMP level-α test for test problem (5.3) is that φ has level α for test problem (5.3). For this, it is sufficient to show that β_φ is non-decreasing, since then $\beta_\varphi(\zeta) \leq \beta_\varphi(\zeta_0) = \alpha$ for $\zeta \leq \zeta_0$ by assumption.

By Corollary 2.55, β_φ is differentiable with derivative

$$\beta'_\varphi(\zeta) = E_\zeta[(T - E_\zeta[T])\,\varphi], \qquad \zeta \in \Xi^*.$$

Hence, we have for all $\zeta \in \Xi^*$ with $c - E_\zeta[T] \geq 0$ that

$$\beta'_\varphi(\zeta) = \int_{(c,\infty)} (t - E_\zeta[T])\,d(P^*_\zeta)^T(t) + \gamma(c - E_\zeta[T])\,P^*_\zeta(T = c) \geq 0,$$

and for all $\zeta \in \Xi^*$ with $c - E_\zeta[T] < 0$

$$\begin{aligned}\beta'_\varphi(\zeta) &\geq \int_{[c,\infty)} (t - E_\zeta[T])\,d(P^*_\zeta)^T(t) \\ &= \int_{(-\infty,\infty)} (t - E_\zeta[T])\,d(P^*_\zeta)^T(t) - \int_{(-\infty,c)} (t - E_\zeta[T])\,d(P^*_\zeta)^T(t) \\ &= -\int_{(-\infty,c)} (t - E_\zeta[T])\,d(P^*_\zeta)^T(t) \geq 0.\end{aligned}$$

The proof of assertion (b) is analogue to that of (a) and therefore omitted. □

Obviously, the UMP tests in Theorem 5.4 can be chosen as non-randomized tests if T has a continuous distribution.

Remark 5.5 The UMP tests in Theorem 5.4 have even strictly monotone power functions on $\{\zeta \in \Xi^* : 0 < \beta_\varphi(\zeta) < 1\}$, which can be seen as follows. Let φ be the UMP test in Theorem 5.4(a), and let $\zeta_1, \zeta_2 \in \Xi^*$ with $\zeta_1 < \zeta_2$ and $\alpha_0 = \beta_\varphi(\zeta_1) \in (0, 1)$. Then, by inspecting the proof of Theorem 5.4(a) and by Lemma 5.3(a), φ also maximizes $E_{\zeta_2}[\psi]$ among all tests ψ with $E_{\zeta_1}[\psi] = \alpha_0$. In particular, by setting $\psi \equiv \alpha_0$, it follows that $E_{\zeta_2}[\varphi] \geq \alpha_0$. Here, if equality would be true, then $\psi \equiv \alpha_0$ would also be a solution of this maximizing problem and Lemma 5.3(a) then would ensure that there exists a constant $k_0 \in \mathbb{R}$ with $f^*_{\zeta_2} = k_0 f^*_{\zeta_1}$ μ-a.e., which would yield $k_0 = 1$ and thus the contradiction $P^*_{\zeta_2} = P^*_{\zeta_1}$. Hence, we have $\beta_\varphi(\zeta_2) = E_{\zeta_2}[\varphi] > \alpha_0 = \beta_\varphi(\zeta_1)$. By the same arguments, the assertion can be shown for the UMP test in Theorem 5.4(b).

Examples: $\mathfrak{poi}(\bullet)$, $\mathcal{N}(\bullet, \sigma_0^2)$

Example 5.6 Let $X_1, \ldots, X_n$ be an iid sample from $P_a = \mathfrak{poi}(a)$ for some $a \in (0, \infty)$, and consider the test problem

$$H_0 : a \leq a_0 \qquad \leftrightarrow \qquad H_1 : a > a_0,$$

for some fixed $a_0 \in (0, \infty)$. By transforming to the canonical representation of $\mathfrak{poi}(\bullet)$ via $P^*_\zeta = P_{\exp\{\zeta\}}$, $\zeta \in \mathbb{R}$, according to Example 2.37, the test problem becomes

$$H_0 : \zeta \leq \zeta_0 \qquad \leftrightarrow \qquad H_1 : \zeta > \zeta_0$$

with $\zeta_0 = \ln(a_0)$. Applying Theorem 5.4(a) to the corresponding product family $\mathcal{P}^{(n)}$ then yields that

$$\varphi(\boldsymbol{x}) = \mathbb{1}_{(c,\infty)}(T_n(\boldsymbol{x})) + \gamma \mathbb{1}_{\{c\}}(T_n(\boldsymbol{x})), \qquad \boldsymbol{x} = (x_1, \ldots, x_n) \in \mathbb{N}_0^n,$$

forms a UMP level-α test for this test problem, where $T_n(\boldsymbol{x}) = \sum_{i=1}^n x_i$, $\boldsymbol{x} \in \mathbb{N}_0^n$, and the constants $c \in \mathbb{R}$ and $\gamma \in [0, 1]$ are determined by the equation

$$\begin{aligned} \alpha &= (P^*_{\zeta_0})^{(n)}(T_n > c) + \gamma\, (P^*_{\zeta_0})^{(n)}(T_n = c) \\ &= P_{a_0}^{(n)}(T_n > c) + \gamma\, P_{a_0}^{(n)}(T_n = c)\,. \end{aligned}$$

By using Example 3.2, the moment generating function of T_n is given by

$$m_{T_n}(b) = m_T^n(b) = \exp\left\{na(e^b - 1)\right\}, \qquad b \in \mathbb{R},$$

where integration is with respect to $P_a^{(n)}$. This yields $T_n \sim P_{na} = \mathfrak{poi}(na)$. Hence, since $0 \leq \gamma \leq 1$, c must be the minimum integer $m \in \mathbb{N}_0$ such that

$$\alpha \geq P_{a_0}^{(n)}(T_n > m) = e^{-na_0} \sum_{j=m+1}^{\infty} \frac{(na_0)^j}{j!},$$

and γ is then already specified as $\gamma = [\alpha - P_{a_0}^{(n)}(T_n > c)]/P_{a_0}^{(n)}(T_n = c)$.

Example 5.7 Let $X_1, \ldots, X_n$ be an iid sample from $\mathcal{N}(\mu, \sigma_0^2)$ for some $\mu \in \mathbb{R}$ and fixed $\sigma_0^2 \in (0, \infty)$, and consider the test problem

$$H_0 : \mu \geq \mu_0 \qquad \leftrightarrow \qquad H_1 : \mu < \mu_0, \tag{5.6}$$

for some fixed $\mu_0 \in \mathbb{R}$. Obviously, the product family $\mathcal{P}^{(n)}$ of $\mathcal{P} = \mathcal{N}(\bullet, \sigma_0^2) = \{\mathcal{N}(\mu, \sigma_0^2) : \mu \in \mathbb{R}\}$ forms an EF with canonical representation

$$f_\mu^{(n)}(\boldsymbol{x}) = C(\mu)\, e^{\mu T_n(\boldsymbol{x})}\, h(\boldsymbol{x}), \qquad \boldsymbol{x} = (x_1, \ldots, x_n) \in \mathbb{R}^n,$$

where $C(\mu) = \exp\{-n\mu^2/(2\sigma_0^2)\}$, $\mu \in \mathbb{R}$, and

$$T_n(\boldsymbol{x}) = \frac{1}{\sigma_0^2}\sum_{i=1}^{n} x_i \quad \text{and} \quad h(\boldsymbol{x}) = \left(\frac{1}{2\pi\sigma_0^2}\right)^{n/2} \exp\left\{-\frac{1}{2\sigma_0^2}\sum_{i=1}^{n} x_i^2\right\}$$

for $\boldsymbol{x} = (x_1, \ldots, x_n) \in \mathbb{R}^n$ (see Example 2.10). Applying Theorem 5.4(b) to the EF $\mathcal{P}^{(n)}$ then yields that

$$\varphi(\boldsymbol{x}) = \mathbb{1}_{(-\infty,c)}(T_n(\boldsymbol{x})), \qquad \boldsymbol{x} = (x_1, \ldots, x_n) \in \mathbb{R}^n,$$

forms a UMP level-α test for test problem (5.6), where the constant $c \in \mathbb{R}$ is determined by

$$P_{\mu_0}^{(n)}(T_n < c) = \alpha .$$

Here, since T_n is continuously distributed, we have set $\gamma = 0$ and thus chosen a non-randomized test. Since $T_n \sim \mathcal{N}(n\mu_0/\sigma_0^2, n/\sigma_0^2)$ under $P_{\mu_0}^{(n)}$, we conclude that c fulfils

$$\frac{c - n\mu_0/\sigma_0^2}{\sqrt{n/\sigma_0^2}} = u_\alpha ,$$

where u_α denotes the α-quantile of the standard normal distribution $\mathcal{N}(0, 1)$. Equivalently, we have

$$c = \sqrt{\frac{n}{\sigma_0^2}}\, u_\alpha + \frac{n\mu_0}{\sigma_0^2} ,$$

and thus, in terms of the arithmetic mean of $x_1, \ldots, x_n$, a representation of φ as

$$\varphi(\boldsymbol{x}) = \mathbb{1}_{\left(-\infty,\mu_0+u_\alpha\sqrt{\sigma_0^2/n}\right)}\left(\frac{1}{n}\sum_{i=1}^{n} x_i\right), \qquad \boldsymbol{x} = (x_1, \ldots, x_n) \in \mathbb{R}^n .$$

This test is commonly known as Gauss test.

5.2 Two-Sided Test Problems

For *two-sided* test problems, a UMP level-α test does not exist, in general; however, optimal tests for these test problems can be established for one-parameter EFs by farther restricting the set Φ of admissible tests, i.e., from all level-α tests to all unbiased level-α tests for the test problem.

Theorem 5.8 *Under the assumptions of Theorem 5.4 a UMPU level-α test for the two-sided test problem*

$$H_0 : \zeta = \zeta_0 \qquad \leftrightarrow \qquad H_1 : \zeta \neq \zeta_0 \tag{5.7}$$

is given by

$$\varphi(x) = \begin{cases} 1, & T(x) < c_1 \ \text{or} \ T(x) > c_2, \\ \gamma_i, & T(x) = c_i, \ i = 1, 2, \\ 0, & c_1 < T(x) < c_2, \end{cases} \qquad \text{for } x \in \mathcal{X}, \tag{5.8}$$

where the constants $c_1, c_2 \in \mathbb{R}$ and $\gamma_1, \gamma_2 \in [0, 1]$ are determined by the equations

$$E_{\zeta_0}[\varphi] = \alpha \qquad \text{and} \qquad E_{\zeta_0}[\varphi T] = \alpha\, E_{\zeta_0}[T].$$

Proof We first show that every unbiased test with level α for test problem (5.7) is contained in the set

$$\Phi = \{\psi : \psi \text{ is test with } E_{\zeta_0}[\psi] = \alpha \text{ and } E_{\zeta_0}[\psi T] = \alpha\, E_{\zeta_0}[T]\}.$$

Let ψ be an unbiased test with level α for test problem (5.7). From Corollary 2.55, we have that the power function $\beta_\psi(\zeta) = E_\zeta[\psi]$, $\zeta \in \Xi^*$, of ψ is continuously differentiable with derivative

$$\beta'_\psi(\zeta) = E_\zeta[\psi T] - E_\zeta[\psi] E_\zeta[T], \qquad \zeta \in \Xi^*.$$

Since unbiasedness of ψ for test problem (5.7) yields that $\beta_\psi(\zeta_0) \leq \alpha$ and $\beta_\psi(\zeta) \geq \alpha$ for $\zeta \in \Xi^* \setminus \{\zeta_0\}$, it necessarily holds that $\beta_\psi(\zeta_0) = \alpha$ by using the continuity of β_ψ. Moreover, unbiasedness of ψ implies that β_ψ has a global minimum at ζ_0. Since ψ is differentiable, it follows that

$$0 = \beta'_\psi(\zeta_0) = E_{\zeta_0}[\psi T] - E_{\zeta_0}[\psi] E_{\zeta_0}[T] = E_{\zeta_0}[\psi T] - \alpha E_{\zeta_0}[T].$$

Hence, $\psi \in \Phi$ is shown.

Next, note that every UMP test in Φ for test problem (5.7) has level α and must be unbiased for test problem (5.7), as a power comparison with the constant test

$\psi \equiv \alpha$ in Φ shows. Hence, it also forms a UMPU level-α test for this test problem. We therefore aim to find a UMP test in Φ for test problem (5.7). For this, we derive a UMP test in Φ for test problem (5.4) with two simple hypotheses, where $\zeta_1 \in \Xi^*$ with $\zeta_1 \neq \zeta_0$ is fixed; this will lead to the test φ as stated and, since φ does not depend on the special value of ζ_1, it is UMP in Φ even for test problem (5.7) by Definition 5.2.

Let $\zeta_1 \in \Xi^*$ with $\zeta_1 \neq \zeta_0$ be fixed. As in the proof of Theorem 5.4, let $h > 0$ without loss of generality. We apply Lemma 5.3 with $n = 2$, $f_0 = f^*_{\zeta_0}$, $f_1 = Tf^*_{\zeta_0}$ and $f_2 = f^*_{\zeta_1}$, $\alpha_0 = \alpha$ and $\alpha_1 = \alpha E_{\zeta_0}[T]$. Here, the condition that $(\alpha, \alpha E_{\zeta_0}[T]) \in int(Q)$ can be verified as follows.

First, by choosing $\psi \equiv \alpha + \varepsilon$ and $\psi \equiv \alpha - \varepsilon$ for a sufficiently small $\varepsilon > 0$, we obtain that

$$(\alpha + \varepsilon, (\alpha + \varepsilon)E_{\zeta_0}[T]) \in Q \qquad \text{and} \qquad (\alpha - \varepsilon, (\alpha - \varepsilon)E_{\zeta_0}[T]) \in Q\,. \tag{5.9}$$

By Lemma 5.3(b) with $n = 1$, $f_0 = f^*_{\zeta_0}$, $f_1 = Tf^*_{\zeta_0}$, and $\alpha_0 = \alpha$, there exists a test φ_1, which maximizes $E_{\zeta_0}[\psi T]$ among all tests ψ with $E_{\zeta_0}[\psi] = \alpha$. In particular, the choice $\psi \equiv \alpha$ yields that $E_{\zeta_0}[\varphi_1 T] \geq \alpha E_{\zeta_0}[T]$. If this would be an equality, $\psi \equiv \alpha$ would also be a solution of the maximizing problem, and Lemma 5.3(a) then would ensure the existence of a constant $k_0 \in \mathbb{R}$ with $T = k_0$ μ-a.e., which cannot be the case. Hence,

$$E_{\zeta_0}[\varphi_1] = \alpha \qquad \text{and} \qquad E_{\zeta_0}[\varphi_1 T] > \alpha E_{\zeta_0}[T]\,. \tag{5.10}$$

By the same arguments, there exists a test φ_2 with $E_{\zeta_0}[\varphi_2] = 1 - \alpha$ and $E_{\zeta_0}[\varphi_2 T] > (1 - \alpha)E_{\zeta_0}[T]$. The test $1 - \varphi_2$ therefore meets

$$E_{\zeta_0}[1 - \varphi_2] = \alpha \qquad \text{and} \qquad E_{\zeta_0}[(1 - \varphi_2)T] < \alpha E_{\zeta_0}[T]\,. \tag{5.11}$$

Equations (5.9)–(5.11) together with the convexity of Q then guarantee that $(\alpha, \alpha E_{\zeta_0}[T]) \in int(Q)$.

Now, applying Lemma 5.3(a, b) yields that there exists a UMP test φ in Φ for test problem (5.4) with

$$\varphi(x) = \begin{cases} 1, & f^*_{\zeta_1}(x) > (k_0 + k_1 T(x))\, f^*_{\zeta_0}(x)\,, \\ 0, & f^*_{\zeta_1}(x) < (k_0 + k_1 T(x))\, f^*_{\zeta_0}(x)\,, \end{cases}$$

$$= \begin{cases} 1, & \frac{C^*(\zeta_1)}{C^*(\zeta_0)} \exp\{(\zeta_1 - \zeta_0)T(x)\} > k_0 + k_1 T(x)\,, \\ 0, & \frac{C^*(\zeta_1)}{C^*(\zeta_0)} \exp\{(\zeta_1 - \zeta_0)T(x)\} < k_0 + k_1 T(x)\,, \end{cases} \qquad \mu\text{-a.e.}\,,$$

with constants $k_0, k_1 \in \mathbb{R}$ such that $\varphi \in \Phi$.

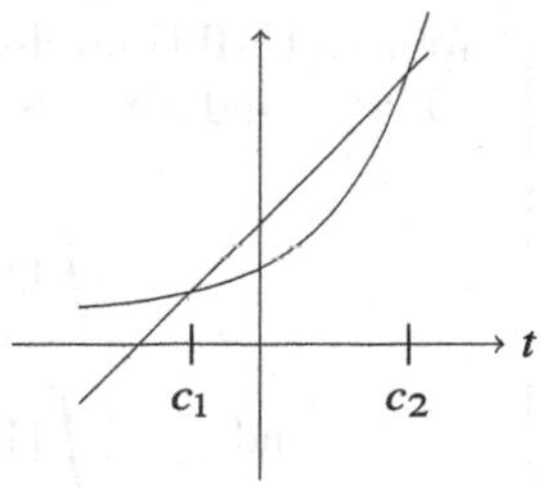

Fig. 5.1 Illustration of the solutions c_1 and c_2 of Eq. (5.12) in t being intersections of a line and a strict convex function

Finally, we consider all solutions of the equation

$$\frac{C^*(\zeta_1)}{C^*(\zeta_0)} e^{(\zeta_1-\zeta_0)t} = k_0 + k_1 t \tag{5.12}$$

with respect to $t \in \mathbb{R}$. If Eq. (5.12) would have no solution in t, then it would follow that $\varphi \equiv 0$ or $\varphi \equiv 1$ in contradiction to $E_{\zeta_0}[\varphi] = \alpha$. On the other hand, since the left-hand side of Eq. (5.12) is strictly convex as a function of t, there exist at most two solutions of Eq. (5.12) in t. φ therefore admits a representation as in formula (5.8) with constants $c_1, c_2 \in \mathbb{R}$ and $\gamma_1, \gamma_2 \in [0, 1]$ such that $\varphi \in \Phi$ ($c_1 = c_2$ and $\gamma_1 = \gamma_2$ if Eq. (5.12) has only one solution). See Fig. 5.1 for an illustration. □

Example: $\mathcal{E}(\bullet)$

Example 5.9 Let $X_1, \ldots, X_n$ be an iid sample from $\mathcal{E}(\lambda) \in \mathcal{P} = \mathcal{E}(\bullet)$ for some $\lambda \in (0, \infty)$, and consider the test problem

$$H_0 : \lambda = \lambda_0 \quad \leftrightarrow \quad H_1 : \lambda \neq \lambda_0 ,$$

for some fixed $\lambda_0 \in \mathbb{R}$. By transforming to the canonical representation of $\mathcal{E}(\bullet)$ via $P_\zeta^* = \mathcal{E}(-1/\zeta)$, $\zeta \in (-\infty, 0)$, according to Example 2.12, the test problem becomes

$$H_0 : \zeta = \zeta_0 \quad \leftrightarrow \quad H_1 : \zeta \neq \zeta_0$$

with $\zeta_0 = -1/\lambda_0$. Applying Theorem 5.8 to the corresponding product family $\mathcal{P}^{(n)}$ then yields that

$$\varphi(\boldsymbol{x}) = 1 - \mathbb{1}_{[c_1,c_2]}(T_n(\boldsymbol{x})) , \qquad \boldsymbol{x} = (x_1, \ldots, x_n) \in (0, \infty)^n ,$$

forms a UMPU level-α test for this test problem, where $T_n(\boldsymbol{x}) = \sum_{i=1}^n x_i$, $\boldsymbol{x} \in (0, \infty)^n$, and the constants $c_1, c_2 \in \mathbb{R}$ are determined by the equations

$$\int [1 - \mathbb{1}_{[c_1,c_2]}(T_n)] \, d(P^*_{\zeta_0})^{(n)} = \alpha$$

$$\text{and} \qquad \int [1 - \mathbb{1}_{[c_1,c_2]}(T_n)] \, T_n \, d(P^*_{\zeta_0})^{(n)} = \alpha \int T_n \, d(P^*_{\zeta_0})^{(n)} .$$

Here, since T_n is continuously distributed, we have set $\gamma_i = 0$, $i = 1, 2$. Moreover, we have that $T_n \sim \mathcal{G}(-1/\zeta_0, n) = \mathcal{G}(\lambda_0, n)$ with corresponding density $f_{\lambda_0,n}$ and mean $n\lambda_0$ under $(P^*_{\zeta_0})^{(n)}$. Hence, we may rewrite the above equations as

$$\int_{c_1}^{c_2} f_{\lambda_0,n}(t) \, dt = 1 - \alpha \qquad \text{and} \qquad \int_{c_1}^{c_2} t \, f_{\lambda_0,n}(t) \, dt = n\lambda_0(1 - \alpha) .$$

It can be shown analytically that these equations have a unique solution in $(c_1, c_2) \in \mathbb{R}^2$, which does not depend on λ_0; for a given sample size n and a desired significance level α, this solution can be obtained numerically, for instance, via the Newton-Raphson method (see, e.g., [7]).

Besides one- and two-sided test problems, choosing a bounded interval as (either null or alternative) hypothesis may also be of interest in applications, which are known as *hypotheses of (non)-equivalence* in the literature (see [62] for an extensive account on the topic). For one-parameter EFs, optimal tests for these test problems can be derived in a similar way as in the proofs of Theorems 5.4 and 5.8. They are stated in the following theorem; a proof can be found, for instance, in [63, Section 2.4].

Theorem 5.10 *Let the assumptions of Theorem 5.4 be given, and let $\zeta_1, \zeta_2 \in \Xi^*$ with $\zeta_1 < \zeta_2$. Then, the following assertions are true:*

(a) For the test problem

$$H_0 : \zeta \in [\zeta_1, \zeta_2] \qquad \leftrightarrow \qquad H_1 : \zeta \notin [\zeta_1, \zeta_2] ,$$

a UMPU level-α- test is given by φ in formula (5.8).

(b) For the test problem

$$H_0 : \zeta \notin (\zeta_1, \zeta_2) \qquad \leftrightarrow \qquad H_1 : \zeta \in (\zeta_1, \zeta_2) ,$$

a UMP level-α test is given by

$$\varphi(x) = \begin{cases} 1, & c_1 < T(x) < c_2, \\ \gamma_i, & T(x) = c_i,\ i = 1, 2, \\ 0, & T(x) < c_1 \text{ or } T(x) > c_2, \end{cases} \qquad \text{for } x \in \mathcal{X}.$$

In (a) and (b), respectively, the constants $c_1, c_2 \in \mathbb{R}$ and $\gamma_1, \gamma_2 \in [0, 1]$ are each determined by the equations

$$E_{\zeta_1}[\varphi] = \alpha \qquad \text{and} \qquad E_{\zeta_2}[\varphi] = \alpha.$$

Remark 5.11 Note that, since every UMP level-α test is unbiased, the tests in Theorems 5.4 and 5.10(b) are also UMPU level-α tests for the given test problem.

5.3 Testing for a Selected Parameter

In multiparameter EFs ($k > 1$), UMPU level-α tests for test problems concerning a single parameter ζ_1, say, may be derived as well. We illustrate the key arguments by considering the regular EF $\mathcal{P} = \{P_{\boldsymbol{\zeta}}^* : \boldsymbol{\zeta} = (\zeta_1, \zeta_2)^t \in \Xi^*\}$ with minimal canonical representation

$$f_{\boldsymbol{\zeta}}^*(x) = C^*(\boldsymbol{\zeta}) \exp\{\zeta_1 T_1(x) + \zeta_2 T_2(x)\}\, h(x), \qquad x \in \mathcal{X}, \tag{5.13}$$

and the test problem (5.1) with $\Xi_0 = \{\boldsymbol{\zeta} \in \Xi^* : \zeta_1 \le \zeta_0\}$ and $\Xi_1 = \{\boldsymbol{\zeta} \in \Xi^* : \zeta_1 > \zeta_0\}$ or, for short,

$$H_0 : \zeta_1 \le \zeta_0 \qquad \leftrightarrow \qquad H_1 : \zeta_1 > \zeta_0, \tag{5.14}$$

where ζ_0 is fixed. Since $\boldsymbol{T} = (T_1, T_2)^t$ is sufficient for $\mathcal{P}$ by Corollary 3.21, we may restrict ourselves to consider tests $\psi = \psi(\boldsymbol{T})$ that depend on x only through $\boldsymbol{T}(x)$.

Let $B = \{\boldsymbol{\zeta} \in \Xi^* : \zeta_1 = \zeta_0\}$ denote the common boundary of Ξ_0 and Ξ_1. Since the power function of any test is continuous by Corollary 2.55, every unbiased test ψ with level α for test problem (5.14) is necessarily *α-similar* on B, i.e.,

$$E_{\boldsymbol{\zeta}}[\psi(\boldsymbol{T})] = \alpha \qquad \text{for all } \boldsymbol{\zeta} \in B. \tag{5.15}$$

Hence, if we find a UMP test among all tests with level α for test problem (5.14) satisfying condition (5.15), then this is also a UMPU level-α test for test problem (5.14), where unbiasedness of the test is obtained by a power comparison with the constant test $\psi \equiv \alpha$.

Next, note that the power function of every test ψ at $\boldsymbol{\zeta} \in \Xi^*$ can be represented as

$$\beta_\psi(\boldsymbol{\zeta}) = E_{\boldsymbol{\zeta}}[\psi(\boldsymbol{T})] = \int\int \psi(t_1, t_2)\, d(P_{\boldsymbol{\zeta}}^*)^{T_1|T_2=t_2}(t_1)\, d(P_{\boldsymbol{\zeta}}^*)^{T_2}(t_2)\,. \tag{5.16}$$

A crucial point is now that T_2 is a sufficient and (boundedly) complete statistic for the EF $\{P_{\boldsymbol{\zeta}}^* : \boldsymbol{\zeta} \in B\}$, which follows by setting $\zeta_1 = \zeta_0$ in formula (5.13) and then applying Corollary 3.21. The tests satisfying condition (5.15) are therefore exactly the tests having so-called *Neyman structure* with respect to T_2, i.e., the tests ψ that meet

$$\int \psi(t_1, t_2)\, d(P_{\boldsymbol{\zeta}}^*)^{T_1|T_2=t_2}(t_1) = \alpha \qquad (P_{\boldsymbol{\zeta}}^*)^{T_2}\text{-a.s.}, \; \boldsymbol{\zeta} \in B$$

(see, for instance, [40, p. 118/119] and [55, pp. 405/406]).

This suggests to consider the inner integral in representation (5.16) separately for every fixed t_2, which reduces the maximizing problem to the one-parameter case, since the conditional distribution of T_1 given $T_2 = t_2$ does not depend on ζ_2 and forms a one-parameter EF in ζ_1 (see Theorem 3.11).

Detailed proofs of the following theorems can be found, e.g., in [40, pp. 119–122] and [55, pp. 406–408]. Without loss of generality, the results are formulated in terms of the first parameter.

Theorem 5.12 *Let $\mathcal{P} = \{P_{\boldsymbol{\zeta}}^* = f_{\boldsymbol{\zeta}}^* \mu : \boldsymbol{\zeta} \in \Xi^*\}$ be a regular EF with minimal canonical representation of the μ-densities given by*

$$f_{\boldsymbol{\zeta}}^*(x) = C^*(\boldsymbol{\zeta}) \exp\{\zeta_1 U(x) + (\zeta_2, \ldots, \zeta_k)\boldsymbol{V}(x)\}\, h(x)\,, \qquad x \in \mathcal{X}\,,$$

for $\boldsymbol{\zeta} = (\zeta_1, \ldots, \zeta_k)^t \in \Xi^* \subset \mathbb{R}^k$, where $U : (\mathcal{X}, \mathcal{B}) \to (\mathbb{R}^1, \mathbb{B}^1)$ is a random variable and $\boldsymbol{V} : (\mathcal{X}, \mathcal{B}) \to (\mathbb{R}^{k-1}, \mathbb{B}^{k-1})$ is a column random vector. Moreover, let $\boldsymbol{\eta} = (\eta_1, \ldots, \eta_k)^t \in \Xi^*$ and $\alpha \in (0, 1)$. Then, we have:

(a) For the one-sided test problem

$$H_0 : \zeta_1 \le \eta_1 \qquad \leftrightarrow \qquad H_1 : \zeta_1 > \eta_1\,,$$

a UMPU level-α test is given by $\varphi = \psi \circ (U, \boldsymbol{V})$ with mapping

$$\psi(u, \boldsymbol{v}) = \mathbb{1}_{(c(\boldsymbol{v}),\infty)}(u) + \gamma(\boldsymbol{v})\, \mathbb{1}_{\{c(\boldsymbol{v})\}}(u)\,, \qquad u \in \mathbb{R}, \; \boldsymbol{v} \in \mathbb{R}^{k-1}\,.$$

(b) For the one-sided test problem

$$H_0 : \zeta_1 \ge \eta_1 \qquad \leftrightarrow \qquad H_1 : \zeta_1 < \eta_1$$

a UMPU level-α test is given by $\varphi = \psi \circ (U, \boldsymbol{V})$ with mapping

$$\psi(u, \boldsymbol{v}) = \mathbb{1}_{(-\infty, c(\boldsymbol{v}))}(u) + \gamma(\boldsymbol{v})\, \mathbb{1}_{\{c(\boldsymbol{v})\}}(u), \qquad u \in \mathbb{R},\ \boldsymbol{v} \in \mathbb{R}^{k-1}.$$

In (a) and (b), respectively, the mappings $c, \gamma : (\mathbb{R}^{k-1}, \mathbb{B}^{k-1}) \to (\mathbb{R}^1, \mathbb{B}^1)$ with $0 \le \gamma \le 1$ are each determined by the equations

$$E_{\eta}[\varphi | \boldsymbol{V} = \boldsymbol{v}] = \alpha, \qquad \boldsymbol{v} \in \mathbb{R}^{k-1}. \tag{5.17}$$

Note that the expected value in formula (5.17) is independent of $\eta_2, \ldots, \eta_k$, since

$$E_{\eta}[\varphi | \boldsymbol{V} = \boldsymbol{v}] = E_{\eta}[\psi(U, \boldsymbol{v}) | \boldsymbol{V} = \boldsymbol{v}] = \int \psi(u, \boldsymbol{v})\, d(P_{\eta}^{*})^{U|\boldsymbol{V}=\boldsymbol{v}}(u),$$

and the conditional distribution of U given $\boldsymbol{V} = \boldsymbol{v}$ under P_{η}^{*} does only depend on η_1.

Theorem 5.13 *Under the assumptions of Theorem 5.12 a UMPU level-α test for the two-sided test problem*

$$H_0 : \zeta_1 = \eta_1 \qquad \leftrightarrow \qquad H_1 : \zeta_1 \neq \eta_1$$

is given by $\varphi = \psi \circ (U, \boldsymbol{V})$ with mapping

$$\psi(u, \boldsymbol{v}) = \begin{cases} 1, & u < c_1(\boldsymbol{v}) \text{ or } u > c_2(\boldsymbol{v}), \\ \gamma_i(\boldsymbol{v}), & u = c_i(\boldsymbol{v}),\ i = 1, 2, \\ 0, & c_1(\boldsymbol{v}) < u < c_2(\boldsymbol{v}), \end{cases} \qquad u \in \mathbb{R}^1,\ \boldsymbol{v} \in \mathbb{R}^{k-1}.$$

Here, the mappings $c_i, \gamma_i : (\mathbb{R}^{k-1}, \mathbb{B}^{k-1}) \to (\mathbb{R}^1, \mathbb{B}^1)$ with $0 \le \gamma_i \le 1$, $i = 1, 2$, are determined by the equations

$$E_{\eta}[\varphi | \boldsymbol{V} = \boldsymbol{v}] = \alpha \quad \text{and} \quad E_{\eta}[\varphi\, U | \boldsymbol{V} = \boldsymbol{v}] = \alpha\, E_{\eta}[U | \boldsymbol{V} = \boldsymbol{v}] \tag{5.18}$$

for $\boldsymbol{v} \in \mathbb{R}^{k-1}$.

The expected values in formula (5.18) are all independent of $\eta_2, \ldots, \eta_k$.

Respective statements hold true for the test problems in Theorem 5.10 with interval hypotheses.

Example: $\mathcal{N}_2(\bullet, \boldsymbol{\Sigma}_0)$

Example 5.14 Let $\mathcal{P} = \mathcal{N}_2(\bullet, \boldsymbol{\Sigma}_0) = \{\mathcal{N}_2(\boldsymbol{\mu}, \boldsymbol{\Sigma}_0) : \boldsymbol{\mu} \in \mathbb{R}^2\}$ be the EF of *bivariate normal distributions* according to Example 2.18 with $k = 2$ and fixed covariance matrix

$$\boldsymbol{\Sigma}_0 = \begin{pmatrix} \sigma_1^2 & \sigma_{12} \\ \sigma_{12} & \sigma_2^2 \end{pmatrix},$$

where $\sigma_1, \sigma_2 > 0$ and $\sigma_{12} \in \mathbb{R}$ with $\sigma_{12}^2 < \sigma_1^2\sigma_2^2$. We assume to have an iid sample $\boldsymbol{X}^{(1)}, \ldots, \boldsymbol{X}^{(n)}$ from $P_{\boldsymbol{\mu}}$ and consider the test problem

$$H_0 : \mu_1 \leq \eta_1 \quad \leftrightarrow \quad H_1 : \mu_1 > \eta_1 \tag{5.19}$$

for fixed $\eta_1 \in \mathbb{R}$. From Example 2.18, we know that $P_{\boldsymbol{\mu}}^{\boldsymbol{T}} = \mathcal{N}_2(\boldsymbol{\Sigma}_0^{-1}\boldsymbol{\mu}, \boldsymbol{\Sigma}_0^{-1})$ for $\boldsymbol{T}(\boldsymbol{x}) = \boldsymbol{\Sigma}_0^{-1}\boldsymbol{x}$, $\boldsymbol{x} \in \mathbb{R}^2$. For the product family $\mathcal{P}^{(n)}$, it therefore follows that $\boldsymbol{T}^{(n)}(\tilde{\boldsymbol{x}}) = \sum_{i=1}^n \boldsymbol{T}(\boldsymbol{x}^{(i)})$, $\tilde{\boldsymbol{x}} = (\boldsymbol{x}^{(1)}, \ldots, \boldsymbol{x}^{(n)}) \in (\mathbb{R}^2)^n$ has a $\mathcal{N}_2(n\boldsymbol{\Sigma}_0^{-1}\boldsymbol{\mu}, n\boldsymbol{\Sigma}_0^{-1})$-distribution under $P_{\boldsymbol{\mu}}^{(n)}$, where

$$n\,\boldsymbol{\Sigma}_0^{-1} = \frac{n}{\sigma_1^2\sigma_2^2 - \sigma_{12}^2} \begin{pmatrix} \sigma_2^2 & -\sigma_{12} \\ -\sigma_{12} & \sigma_1^2 \end{pmatrix} = \begin{pmatrix} \tau_1^2 & \tau_{12} \\ \tau_{12} & \tau_2^2 \end{pmatrix}, \quad \text{say}. \tag{5.20}$$

The conditional distribution of $T_1^{(n)}$ given $T_2^{(n)} = v$ under $P_{\boldsymbol{\mu}}^{(n)}$ is a univariate normal distribution with mean $\mu(v)$ and variance $\sigma^2(v)$ given by

$$\begin{aligned} \mu(v) &= \tau_1^2\mu_1 + \tau_{12}\mu_2 + \frac{\tau_1}{\tau_2}\left(\frac{\tau_{12}}{\tau_1\tau_2}\right)\left[v - (\tau_{12}\mu_1 + \tau_2^2\mu_2)\right] \\ &= \tau_1^2\mu_1 + \tau_{12}\mu_2 + \frac{\tau_{12}}{\tau_2^2}\left(v - \tau_{12}\mu_1 - \tau_2^2\mu_2\right) \\ &= \frac{1}{\tau_2^2}\left(\tau_1^2\tau_2^2 - \tau_{12}^2\right)\mu_1 + \frac{\tau_{12}}{\tau_2^2}v = \frac{n\mu_1 - \sigma_{12}v}{\sigma_1^2} \end{aligned}$$

and $$\sigma^2(v) = \left(1 - \frac{\tau_{12}^2}{\tau_1^2\tau_2^2}\right)\tau_1^2 = \frac{1}{\tau_2^2}\left(\tau_1^2\tau_2^2 - \tau_{12}^2\right) = \frac{n}{\sigma_1^2},$$

where the latter is free of v. In the derivation, we have used the identity

$$\tau_1^2\tau_2^2 - \tau_{12}^2 = \frac{n^2}{\sigma_1^2\sigma_2^2 - \sigma_{12}^2},$$

which is obtained by considering determinants in formula (5.20), as well as the equations $\tau_{12}/\tau_2^2 = -\sigma_{12}/\sigma_1^2$ and $\tau_2^2 = n\sigma_1^2/(\sigma_1^2\sigma_2^2 - \sigma_{12}^2)$. Note that the conditional distribution does not depend on μ_2. Denoting by $c_{1-\alpha}(v)$ the $(1-\alpha)$-quantile of this distribution, it holds for $v \in \mathbb{R}$ that

$$u_{1-\alpha} = \frac{c_{1-\alpha}(v) - \mu(v)}{\sigma(v)}$$

and thus $$c_{1-\alpha}(v) = u_{1-\alpha}\,\sigma(v) + \mu(v) = u_{1-\alpha}\sqrt{\frac{n}{\sigma_1^2}} + \frac{n\mu_1 - \sigma_{12}v}{\sigma_1^2},$$

where $u_{1-\alpha}$ is the $(1-\alpha)$-quantile of the standard normal distribution $\mathcal{N}(0, 1)$. Hence, by Theorem 5.12(a), a UMPU level-α test for test problem (5.19) is given by

$$\varphi(\tilde{\boldsymbol{x}}) = \mathbb{1}_{(c(T_2^{(n)}(\tilde{\boldsymbol{x}})),\infty)}(T_1^{(n)}(\tilde{\boldsymbol{x}}))\,, \qquad \tilde{\boldsymbol{x}} \in (\mathbb{R}^2)^n\,,$$

with $$c(v) = u_{1-\alpha}\sqrt{\frac{n}{\sigma_1^2}} + \frac{n\eta_1 - \sigma_{12}v}{\sigma_1^2}\,, \qquad v \in \mathbb{R}\,.$$

5.4 Testing for Several Parameters

In the preceding sections, we have proposed optimal tests for test problems concerning a single parameter of a one- or multiparameter EF. Here, we consider tests for test problem (5.1) with parameter set $\Xi_0 \subset \mathbb{R}^k$ making assumptions on more than one component of $\boldsymbol{\zeta}$, where we focus on likelihood-ratio tests. On the one hand, these tests enable to check conjectures on several parameters simultaneously as, for instance, a simple null hypothesis by choosing $\Xi_0 = \{\boldsymbol{\eta}\}$ for some fixed $\boldsymbol{\eta} \in \Xi$. On the other hand, they may be used to test for relations between the parameters; a homogeneity test, for example, is obtained by setting $\Xi_0 = \{\boldsymbol{\zeta} \in \Xi : \zeta_1 = \cdots = \zeta_k\}$.

Definition 5.15 Let μ be a σ-finite measure and $\mathcal{P} = \{f_{\boldsymbol{\zeta}}^* \mu : \boldsymbol{\zeta} \in \Xi\}$, $\Xi \subset \mathbb{R}^k$, be a family of probability distributions on a measurable space $(\mathcal{X}, \mathcal{B})$. Moreover, let $\emptyset \neq \Xi_0 \subsetneq \Xi$ and $\alpha \in (0, 1)$. For the test problem

$$H_0 : \boldsymbol{\zeta} \in \Xi_0 \quad \leftrightarrow \quad H_1 : \boldsymbol{\zeta} \in \Xi \setminus \Xi_0\,, \tag{5.21}$$

(continued)

Definition 5.15 (continued)
the *likelihood-ratio (LR) test* with level α is defined as

$$\varphi_\Lambda(x) = \mathbb{1}_{(c,\infty)}(\Lambda(x)) + \gamma\,\mathbb{1}_{\{c\}}(\Lambda(x)), \qquad x \in \mathcal{X},$$

provided that the test statistic

$$\Lambda(x) = -2\,\ln\left(\frac{\sup_{\zeta\in\Xi_0} f_\zeta^*(x)}{\sup_{\zeta\in\Xi} f_\zeta^*(x)}\right), \qquad x \in \mathcal{X},$$

is well-defined μ-a.e.. Here, the constants $c \geq 0$ and $\gamma \in [0,1]$ are determined by the equation

$$\sup_{\zeta\in\Xi_0} E_\zeta[\varphi_\Lambda] = \alpha\,.$$

The LR test compares the maximum 'probability' $f_\zeta^*(x)$ of observing x under Ξ_0 with the one under Ξ; the null hypothesis is then rejected if the ratio of both values is (too) small (see the representations of Λ and φ_Λ in Definition 5.15). The numerator and denominator in the expression of Λ are nothing but the density $f_\zeta^*(x)$, where the parameter is chosen as the ML estimate of $\boldsymbol{\zeta}$ in Ξ_0 and in Ξ, respectively.

In minimal regular EFs, Λ is closely related to the Kullback-Leibler divergence.

Theorem 5.16 *Let $\mathcal{P}$ be a regular EF with minimal canonical representation (4.1), and let x be a realization of the random variable X with distribution $P_\zeta^* \in \mathcal{P}$. If the ML estimate $\hat{\boldsymbol{\zeta}}(x)$ of $\boldsymbol{\zeta}$ in Ξ^* and the ML estimate $\hat{\boldsymbol{\zeta}}_0(x)$ of $\boldsymbol{\zeta}$ in Ξ_0 based on x exist, then the test statistic of the LR test for test problem (5.21) with $\Xi = \Xi^*$ is given by*

$$\Lambda(x) = 2\,D_{KL}(\hat{\boldsymbol{\zeta}}(x), \Xi_0) = 2\,D_{KL}(\hat{\boldsymbol{\zeta}}(x), \hat{\boldsymbol{\zeta}}_0(x))\,, \qquad (5.22)$$

$$\textit{where} \qquad D_{KL}(\boldsymbol{\zeta}, \Xi_0) = \inf_{\boldsymbol{\eta}\in\Xi_0} D_{KL}(\boldsymbol{\zeta}, \boldsymbol{\eta})\,, \qquad \boldsymbol{\zeta} \in \Xi^*\,.$$

Proof Without loss of generality, we assume that $h(x) > 0$. Then, since the logarithm is strictly increasing, we have

$$\begin{aligned}\Lambda(x) &= 2\,[\ln(f_{\hat{\boldsymbol{\zeta}}(x)}^*(x)) - \ln(\sup_{\boldsymbol{\zeta}\in\Xi_0} f_{\boldsymbol{\zeta}}^*(x))] \\ &= 2\left(\hat{\boldsymbol{\zeta}}(x)^t\boldsymbol{T}(x) - \kappa(\hat{\boldsymbol{\zeta}}(x)) - \sup_{\boldsymbol{\zeta}\in\Xi_0}\{\boldsymbol{\zeta}^t\boldsymbol{T}(x) - \kappa(\boldsymbol{\zeta})\}\right)\end{aligned}$$

$$= 2 \inf_{\zeta \in \Xi_0} \left(\hat{\xi}(x)^t T(x) - \kappa(\hat{\xi}(x)) - (\zeta^t T(x) - \kappa(\zeta)) \right)$$

$$= 2 \inf_{\zeta \in \Xi_0} \left(\kappa(\zeta) - \kappa(\hat{\xi}(x)) + (\hat{\xi}(x) - \zeta)^t T(x) \right)$$

Now, by Theorem 4.3, $T(x) = \pi(\hat{\xi}(x))$, and the first equality in formula (5.22) follows from Lemma 3.37. Since the supremum of $\zeta^t T(x) - \kappa(\zeta)$, $\zeta \in \Xi_0$, is attained at $\hat{\xi}_0(x)$, the equation $\Lambda(x) = 2D_{KL}(\hat{\xi}(x), \hat{\xi}_0(x))$ is also valid. □

In particular, for fixed $\eta \in \Xi^*$ and the test problem

$$H_0 : \zeta = \eta \quad \leftrightarrow \quad H_1 : \zeta \neq \eta , \tag{5.23}$$

with a simple null hypothesis, Theorem 5.16 yields that $\Lambda = 2D_{KL}(\hat{\xi}, \eta)$ provided that the ML estimate $\hat{\xi}(x)$ of ζ exists for $x \in \mathcal{X}$.

Remark 5.17 The EF structure may also be useful for deriving other well known test statistics for multivariate test problems. For test problem (5.21), if all appearing quantities exist, the *Rao score statistic* and the *Wald statistic* are defined as

$$R = U_{\hat{\xi}_0}^t \, \mathbf{I}(\hat{\xi}_0)^{-1} \, U_{\hat{\xi}_0}$$

$$\text{and} \qquad W = g(\hat{\xi})^t \, [\mathbf{D}_g(\hat{\xi}) \, \mathbf{I}(\hat{\xi})^{-1} \, \mathbf{D}_g(\hat{\xi})^t]^{-1} \, g(\hat{\xi}) ,$$

where U_ζ is the score statistic and $\mathbf{I}(\zeta)$ is the Fisher information matrix at ζ, and $g : \Xi \to \mathbb{R}^q$, $q \leq k$, is a differentiable function with Jacobian matrix $\mathbf{D}_g(\zeta)$ of full rank q at every $\zeta \in \Xi$, which satisfies that $g(\zeta) = \mathbf{0}$ if and only if $\zeta \in \Xi_0$ (see, e.g., [53, pp. 239/240]). Note that R does only depend on the MLE $\hat{\xi}_0$ of ζ in Ξ_0, whereas W only depends on the MLE $\hat{\xi}$ of ζ in Ξ. The *Rao score test* and the *Wald test* then reject H_0 for (too) large values of R and W, respectively. These decision rules are based on the fact that, if $\zeta \in \Xi_0$ is true, then, on the one hand, $U_{\hat{\xi}_0}$ will tend to be close to $U_{\hat{\xi}} = \mathbf{0}$ and, on the other hand, $g(\hat{\xi})$ is expected to be small as an estimator of $g(\zeta) = \mathbf{0}$. Now, if the underlying model forms a minimal regular EF, we may utilize the representations for U_ζ and $\mathbf{I}(\zeta)$ as derived in Theorem 3.29 and make also use of the results in Sects. 4.1 and 4.2 to find the MLEs $\hat{\xi}$ and $\hat{\xi}_0$.

Example: $\mathcal{N}_k(\bullet, \mathbf{\Sigma}_0)$

Example 5.18 Let $X^{(1)}, \ldots, X^{(n)}$ be an iid sample from $\mathcal{N}_k(\mu, \mathbf{\Sigma}_0)$ for some $\mu \in \mathbb{R}^k$ and fixed $\mathbf{\Sigma}_0 \in \mathbb{R}^{k \times k}$ with $\mathbf{\Sigma}_0 > 0$, and consider the test problem

$$H_0 : \mu = \eta \quad \leftrightarrow \quad H_1 : \mu \neq \eta , \tag{5.24}$$

for some fixed $\boldsymbol{\eta} \in \mathbb{R}^k$. From Example 4.10, the ML estimate of $\boldsymbol{\mu}$ based on realizations $\boldsymbol{x}^{(1)}, \ldots, \boldsymbol{x}^{(n)}$ of $\boldsymbol{X}^{(1)}, \ldots, \boldsymbol{X}^{(n)}$ is given by $\hat{\boldsymbol{\mu}}^{(n)}(\boldsymbol{x}^{(1)}, \ldots, \boldsymbol{x}^{(n)}) = \sum_{i=1}^{n} \boldsymbol{x}^{(i)}/n$. Hence, by using Theorem 5.16 and the representation of D_{KL} derived in Example 3.41, the test statistic of the LR test for test problem (5.24) is given by

$$\Lambda_n = 2\, n\, D_{KL}(\hat{\boldsymbol{\mu}}^{(n)}, \boldsymbol{\eta}) = n\, ||\hat{\boldsymbol{\mu}}^{(n)} - \boldsymbol{\eta}||^2_{\boldsymbol{\Sigma}_0} .$$

Here, note that nD_{KL} is the Kullback-Leibler divergence corresponding to the EF $\mathcal{P}^{(n)}$ of product measures. Under H_0, we have

$$\boldsymbol{\Sigma}_0^{-1/2} \sqrt{n} \left(\hat{\boldsymbol{\mu}}^{(n)} - \boldsymbol{\eta} \right) \sim \mathcal{N}_k(\mathbf{0}, \mathbf{E}_k) ,$$

where $\mathbf{E}_k$ is the k-dimensional unit matrix and $\boldsymbol{\Sigma}_0^{-1/2} \in \mathbb{R}^{k\times k}$ is a matrix satisfying $\boldsymbol{\Sigma}_0^{-1/2} > 0$ and $\boldsymbol{\Sigma}_0^{-1/2}\boldsymbol{\Sigma}_0^{-1/2} = \boldsymbol{\Sigma}_0^{-1}$, the existence of which is ensured by the spectral theorem. Thus, under H_0, $\Lambda_n \sim \chi^2(k)$, i.e., Λ_n has a chi-square distribution with k degrees of freedom. The LR test with level α is therefore given by

$$\varphi(\tilde{\boldsymbol{x}}) = \mathbb{1}_{(\chi^2_{1-\alpha}(k),\infty)} \left(n\, ||\hat{\boldsymbol{\mu}}(\tilde{\boldsymbol{x}}) - \boldsymbol{\eta}||^2_{\boldsymbol{\Sigma}_0} \right) , \qquad \tilde{\boldsymbol{x}} = (\boldsymbol{x}^{(1)}, \ldots, \boldsymbol{x}^{(n)}) \in (\mathbb{R}^k)^n ,$$

where $\chi^2_{1-\alpha}(k)$ denotes the $(1-\alpha)$-quantile of $\chi^2(k)$ (see, e.g., [45, p. 124]).

Now, let us derive the Rao score statistic and the Wald statistic for test problem (5.24) as introduced in Remark 5.17, where we choose $g(\boldsymbol{\mu}) = \boldsymbol{\mu} - \boldsymbol{\eta}$, $\boldsymbol{\mu} \in \mathbb{R}^k$. First, note that by Example 2.18 and Theorem 3.13(b) the statistic $\boldsymbol{T}^{(n)}$ for the product EF $\mathcal{P}^{(n)}$ can be represented as $\boldsymbol{T}^{(n)} = n\boldsymbol{\Sigma}_0^{-1}\hat{\mu}^{(n)}$. According to Theorem 3.29 and Example 3.35, the score statistic and the Fisher information matrix belonging to $\mathcal{P}^{(n)}$ are therefore given by $\boldsymbol{U}_{\boldsymbol{\mu}}^{(n)} = n\boldsymbol{\Sigma}_0^{-1}(\hat{\boldsymbol{\mu}}^{(n)} - \boldsymbol{\mu})$ and $\mathbf{I}^{(n)}(\boldsymbol{\mu}) = n\boldsymbol{\Sigma}_0^{-1}$ for $\boldsymbol{\mu} \in \mathbb{R}^k$. Hence, the Rao score statistic is

$$R_n = [\boldsymbol{U}_{\boldsymbol{\eta}}^{(n)}]^t\, [\mathbf{I}^{(n)}(\boldsymbol{\eta})]^{-1}\, \boldsymbol{U}_{\boldsymbol{\eta}}^{(n)} = n\, ||\hat{\boldsymbol{\mu}}^{(n)} - \boldsymbol{\eta}||^2_{\boldsymbol{\Sigma}_0} .$$

Moreover, we have $\mathbf{D}_g(\boldsymbol{\mu}) = \mathbf{E}_k$, $\boldsymbol{\mu} \in \mathbb{R}^k$, and the Wald statistic is

$$W_n = g(\hat{\boldsymbol{\mu}}^{(n)})^t\, \mathbf{I}^{(n)}(\hat{\boldsymbol{\mu}}^{(n)})\, g(\hat{\boldsymbol{\mu}}^{(n)}) = n\, ||\hat{\boldsymbol{\mu}}^{(n)} - \boldsymbol{\eta}||^2_{\boldsymbol{\Sigma}_0} .$$

Hence, in the actual case, all three test statistics Λ_n, R_n, and W_n coincide and thus yield the same test.

In general, for finite sample size $n \in \mathbb{N}$, the distribution of Λ_n under the null hypothesis is not explicitly available. However, for sufficiently large n, we may employ the asymptotic distribution of Λ_n under H_0 instead, which is easily derived by using the properties of the EF. Choosing the $(1-\alpha)$-quantile of the asymptotic distribution as critical value for Λ_n, the actual level of the test φ_{Λ_n} will converge to the nominal level α, when n tends to infinity.

For a simple null hypothesis, the asymptotic distribution of Λ_n can be obtained from a Taylor series expansion of the log-likelihood function and by using (asymptotic) properties of the MLE of $\boldsymbol{\zeta}$ (see, e.g., [54, pp. 151–156]).

Theorem 5.19 *Let $\mathcal{P}$ be a regular EF with minimal canonical representation (4.1), and let $X^{(1)}, X^{(2)}, \ldots$ be a sequence of iid random variables with distribution $P^*_{\boldsymbol{\zeta}} \in \mathcal{P}$. Moreover, for eventually all $n \in \mathbb{N}$, let the MLE $\hat{\boldsymbol{\zeta}}^{(n)}$ of $\boldsymbol{\zeta}$ in Ξ^* based on $X^{(1)}, \ldots, X^{(n)}$ exist and $\Lambda_n = \Lambda_n(X^{(1)}, \ldots, X^{(n)})$ denote the test statistic of the LR test for test problem (5.23) based on $X^{(1)}, \ldots, X^{(n)}$. Then, under H_0,*

$$\Lambda_n \xrightarrow{d} \chi^2(k)$$

for $n \to \infty$, i.e., Λ_n is asymptotically chi-square distributed with k degrees of freedom if n tends to infinity.

Proof Without loss of generality, let $\hat{\boldsymbol{\zeta}}^{(n)}$ exist for all $n \in \mathbb{N}$. Let $\ell_n(\boldsymbol{\zeta}) = \ln(\prod_{i=1}^n f^*_{\boldsymbol{\zeta}}(X^{(i)}))$, $\boldsymbol{\zeta} \in \Xi^*$, denote the log-likelihood function based on $X^{(1)}, \ldots, X^{(n)}$ for $n \in \mathbb{N}$. Moreover, suppose that H_0 is true, i.e., $\boldsymbol{\zeta} = \boldsymbol{\eta}$. Since ℓ_n has a maximum at $\hat{\boldsymbol{\zeta}}^{(n)}$ and Ξ^* is open, it necessarily holds that $\nabla \ell_n(\hat{\boldsymbol{\zeta}}^{(n)}) = 0$ for all $n \in \mathbb{N}$. Hence, the Taylor series expansion of ℓ_n about $\hat{\boldsymbol{\zeta}}^{(n)}$ at $\boldsymbol{\zeta}$ is given by

$$\ell_n(\boldsymbol{\zeta}) = \ell_n(\hat{\boldsymbol{\zeta}}^{(n)}) + \frac{1}{2}(\hat{\boldsymbol{\zeta}}^{(n)} - \boldsymbol{\zeta})^t \, \mathbf{H}_{\ell_n}(\tilde{\boldsymbol{\zeta}}^{(n)})\,(\hat{\boldsymbol{\zeta}}^{(n)} - \boldsymbol{\zeta}),$$

where $\tilde{\boldsymbol{\zeta}}^{(n)}$ is a convex combination of $\boldsymbol{\zeta}$ and $\hat{\boldsymbol{\zeta}}^{(n)}$, $n \in \mathbb{N}$. For the test statistic $\Lambda_n = \Lambda_n(X^{(1)}, \ldots, X^{(n)})$ of the LR test based on $X^{(1)}, \ldots, X^{(n)}$, we thus obtain

$$\begin{aligned}\Lambda_n &= -2\,(\ell_n(\boldsymbol{\zeta}) - \ell_n(\hat{\boldsymbol{\zeta}}^{(n)})) \\ &= \sqrt{n}\,(\hat{\boldsymbol{\zeta}}^{(n)} - \boldsymbol{\zeta})^t \left[-\frac{1}{n}\mathbf{H}_{\ell_n}(\tilde{\boldsymbol{\zeta}}^{(n)})\right] \sqrt{n}(\hat{\boldsymbol{\zeta}}^{(n)} - \boldsymbol{\zeta}).\end{aligned}$$

From Corollary 3.30 and Theorem 2.56, we have that

$$-\frac{1}{n}\mathbf{H}_{\ell_n}(\boldsymbol{\zeta}) = \mathbf{H}_{\kappa}(\boldsymbol{\zeta}) = \mathbf{I}(\boldsymbol{\zeta}) > 0, \qquad \boldsymbol{\zeta} \in \Xi^*,$$

which allows for the representation

$$\Lambda_n = ||\,\mathbf{I}(\tilde{\boldsymbol{\zeta}}^{(n)})^{1/2}\sqrt{n}(\hat{\boldsymbol{\zeta}}^{(n)} - \boldsymbol{\zeta})||_2^2, \tag{5.25}$$

with a matrix $\mathbf{I}(\tilde{\boldsymbol{\zeta}}^{(n)})^{1/2} > 0$ satisfying $\mathbf{I}(\tilde{\boldsymbol{\zeta}}^{(n)})^{1/2}\mathbf{I}(\tilde{\boldsymbol{\zeta}}^{(n)})^{1/2} = \mathbf{I}(\tilde{\boldsymbol{\zeta}}^{(n)})$ for $n \in \mathbb{N}$; here, existence of such a matrix is guaranteed by the spectral theorem. From Theorem 4.31, we have that $\hat{\boldsymbol{\zeta}}^{(n)} \to \boldsymbol{\zeta}$ $\mathbb{P}_{\boldsymbol{\zeta}}$-a.s. and thus also $\tilde{\boldsymbol{\zeta}}^{(n)} \to \boldsymbol{\zeta}$ $\mathbb{P}_{\boldsymbol{\zeta}}$-a.s. for $n \to \infty$. Since the mapping $\mathbf{I}(\cdot)^{1/2}$ is continuous on Ξ^*, it follows that $\mathbf{I}(\tilde{\boldsymbol{\zeta}}^{(n)})^{1/2} \to \mathbf{I}(\boldsymbol{\zeta})^{1/2}$ $\mathbb{P}_{\boldsymbol{\zeta}}$-a.s. for $n \to \infty$. Moreover, by Theorem 4.34,

$$\sqrt{n}\,(\hat{\boldsymbol{\zeta}}^{(n)} - \boldsymbol{\zeta}) \xrightarrow{d} \boldsymbol{N} \sim \mathcal{N}_k(\mathbf{0}, [\mathbf{I}(\boldsymbol{\zeta})]^{-1}),$$

and we conclude from the multivariate Slutsky theorem that

$$\mathbf{I}(\tilde{\boldsymbol{\zeta}}^{(n)})^{1/2}\sqrt{n}(\hat{\boldsymbol{\zeta}}^{(n)} - \boldsymbol{\zeta}) \xrightarrow{d} \mathbf{I}(\boldsymbol{\zeta})^{1/2}\boldsymbol{N} \sim \mathcal{N}_k(\mathbf{0}, \mathbf{E}_k),$$

where $\mathbf{E}_k \in \mathbb{R}^{k \times k}$ denotes the k-dimensional unit matrix. In virtue of the continuous mapping $||\cdot||_2^2$, the assertion now follows from formula (5.25) together with the continuous mapping theorem (see, e.g., [18, Chapter 1, Section 5]). □

Theorem 5.19 is a special case of the following, more general result; its proof can be found, for instance, in [53, p. 240] and [54, pp. 156–160].

Theorem 5.20 *In the situation of Theorem 5.19, let the test problem be replaced by test problem (5.21) with* $\Xi = \Xi^*$ *and*

$$\Xi_0 = \{\boldsymbol{\zeta} \in \Xi^* : g(\boldsymbol{\zeta}) = \mathbf{0}\},$$

where $g : \Xi^* \to \mathbb{R}^q$, $q \le k$, *is a differentiable function with Jacobian matrix* $\mathbf{D}_g(\boldsymbol{\zeta})$ *of full rank q at every* $\boldsymbol{\zeta} \in \Xi^*$. *If the MLE* $\hat{\boldsymbol{\zeta}}_0^{(n)}$ *of* $\boldsymbol{\zeta}$ *in* Ξ_0 *based on* $X^{(1)}, \ldots, X^{(n)}$ *exists for eventually all* $n \in \mathbb{N}$, *then*

$$\Lambda_n \xrightarrow{d} \chi^2(q)$$

under H_0 *for* $n \to \infty$.

The function g in Theorem 5.20 characterizes the null hypothesis in the same way as in Remark 5.17 for the Wald test. Setting $g(\boldsymbol{\zeta}) = \boldsymbol{\zeta} - \boldsymbol{\eta}$, $\boldsymbol{\zeta} \in \Xi^*$, in Theorem 5.20 gives the result of Theorem 5.19. The choice

$$g(\boldsymbol{\zeta}) = (\zeta_{i_1} - \eta_{i_1}, \ldots, \zeta_{i_q} - \eta_{i_q})^t, \qquad \boldsymbol{\zeta} \in \Xi^*,$$

for fixed $\boldsymbol{\eta} = (\eta_1, \ldots, \eta_k)^t \in \Xi^*$ and $i_1, \ldots, i_q \in \{1, \ldots, k\}$ with $i_1 < \cdots < i_q$ corresponds to the null hypothesis $H_0 : \zeta_{i_j} = \eta_{i_j}$ *for all* $1 \le j \le q$, which may therefore be used to check only for particular components of $\boldsymbol{\zeta}$. Moreover, we may test for homogeneity of the parameters, i.e., for $H_0 : \zeta_1 = \cdots = \zeta_k$, by defining, e.g.,

$$g(\boldsymbol{\zeta}) = (\zeta_2 - \zeta_1, \ldots, \zeta_k - \zeta_{k-1})^t , \qquad \boldsymbol{\zeta} \in \Xi^* ,$$

in the case of which $\Lambda_n \xrightarrow{d} \chi^2(k-1)$ under H_0 for $n \to \infty$.

Remark 5.21 Let the iid setup and the test problem in Theorem 5.20 be given. If the respective estimators $\hat{\boldsymbol{\zeta}}_0^{(n)}$ and $\hat{\boldsymbol{\zeta}}^{(n)}$ exist for eventually all $n \in \mathbb{N}$, the Rao score statistic R_n and the Wald statistic W_n (defined on $\mathcal{X}^n$ according to Remark 5.17) are asymptotically $\chi^2(q)$-distributed under H_0 for $n \to \infty$. For the proofs, see, e.g., [53, p. 240] and [54, pp. 156–160].

For further reading on testing hypotheses in EFs, we refer to, for example, [63, 20, 40, 42, 34].

Chapter 6
Exemplary Multivariate Applications

In this chapter, we demonstrate the usefulness of the proposed results for EFs by means of three multivariate examples of different kind. First, for the discrete case, the family of negative multinomial distributions is considered. Then, we turn to the continuous case and study properties of Dirichlet distributions. Finally, the results are applied to joint distributions of generalized order statistics, which form a unifying approach to various models of ordered random variables. In the joint density function of generalized order statistics, an absolutely continuous baseline distribution function can be arbitrarily chosen.

6.1 Negative Multinomial Distribution

The negative multinomial distribution is a natural multivariate extension of the negative binomial distribution (see, for example, [28, Chapter 36]). Suppose that we have an experiment with $k+1$ possible outcomes $O_1, \ldots, O_{k+1}$, which is independently repeated until a given number r of a particular outcome O_{k+1}, say, is observed. Then, the negative multinomial distribution describes the probabilities of observing exactly x_i times outcome O_i for $1 \leq i \leq k$ up to the r-th observation of O_{k+1}.

Definition 6.1 The *negative multinomial distribution* $\mathrm{nm}(r, \boldsymbol{p})$ with $r \in \mathbb{N}$ and $\boldsymbol{p} = (p_1, \ldots, p_k)^t \in (0,1)^k$, $k \in \mathbb{N}$, satisfying $\sum_{j=1}^{k} p_j < 1$ is defined

(continued)

S. Bedbur, U. Kamps, *Multivariate Exponential Families: A Concise Guide to Statistical Inference*, SpringerBriefs in Statistics,
https://doi.org/10.1007/978-3-030-81900-2_6

Definition 6.1 (continued)
as the probability distribution on $\mathbb{N}_0^k$ with counting density

$$f_{\boldsymbol{p}}(\boldsymbol{x}) = \frac{\left(r-1+\sum_{j=1}^k x_j\right)!}{(r-1)!\prod_{j=1}^k x_j!}\left(\prod_{j=1}^k p_j^{x_j}\right)\left(1-\sum_{j=1}^k p_j\right)^r, \qquad (6.1)$$

for $\boldsymbol{x} = (x_1, \ldots, x_k)^t \in \mathbb{N}_0^k$.

The negative multinomial distribution is a member of the more general family of multivariate power series distributions introduced in Remark 2.9.

Rewriting density function (6.1) as

$$f_{\boldsymbol{p}}(\boldsymbol{x}) = C(\boldsymbol{p}) \exp\left\{\sum_{j=1}^k Z_j(\boldsymbol{p})T_j(\boldsymbol{x})\right\} h(\boldsymbol{x}), \qquad \boldsymbol{x} = (x_1, \ldots, x_k)^t \in \mathbb{N}_0^k,$$

with $Z_j(\boldsymbol{p}) = \ln(p_j)$, $1 \leq j \leq k$, and

$$C(\boldsymbol{p}) = \left(1-\sum_{j=1}^k p_j\right)^r,$$

and $T_j(\boldsymbol{x}) = x_j$, $1 \leq j \leq k$, and

$$h(\boldsymbol{x}) = \frac{\left(r-1+\sum_{j=1}^k x_j\right)!}{(r-1)!\prod_{j=1}^k x_j!}, \qquad \boldsymbol{x} = (x_1, \ldots, x_k)^t \in \mathbb{N}_0^k, \qquad (6.2)$$

we directly find that, for fixed $r = r_0 \in \mathbb{N}$, $\mathfrak{nm}(r_0, \bullet) = \{\mathfrak{nm}(r_0, \boldsymbol{p}) : \boldsymbol{p} \in \Theta\}$ forms an EF with parameter space

$$\Theta = \left\{(p_1, \ldots, p_k)^t \in (0,1)^k : \sum_{j=1}^k p_j < 1\right\}.$$

Aiming for inferential results for the negative multinomial distribution, we turn to a minimal canonical representation of $\mathfrak{nm}(r_0, \bullet)$.

Theorem 6.2 *Let $\mathcal{P} = \mathfrak{nm}(r_0, \bullet)$ for some fixed $r_0 \in \mathbb{N}$ as introduced above. Then, we find:*

(a) $ord(\mathcal{P}) = k$.

(b) The natural parameter space of $\mathcal{P}$ is given by

$$\Xi^* = \left\{ \boldsymbol{\zeta} = (\zeta_1, \ldots, \zeta_k)^t \in (-\infty, 0)^k : \sum_{j=1}^{k} e^{\zeta_j} < 1 \right\} .$$

(c) $\mathcal{P}$ is regular with minimal canonical representation given by the counting densities

$$f_{\boldsymbol{\zeta}}^*(\boldsymbol{x}) = \frac{dP_{\boldsymbol{\zeta}}^*}{d\mu_{\mathbb{N}_0^k}}(\boldsymbol{x}) = e^{\boldsymbol{\zeta}^t \boldsymbol{T}(\boldsymbol{x}) - \kappa(\boldsymbol{\zeta})}\, h(\boldsymbol{x}), \qquad \boldsymbol{x} \in \mathbb{N}_0^k, \tag{6.3}$$

for $\boldsymbol{\zeta} \in \Xi^*$, where $\boldsymbol{T}(\boldsymbol{x}) = \boldsymbol{x}$, $\boldsymbol{x} \in \mathbb{N}_0^k$, h is as in formula (6.2), and the cumulant function is given by

$$\kappa(\boldsymbol{\zeta}) = -r_0 \ln\left(1 - \sum_{j=1}^{k} e^{\zeta_j}\right), \qquad \boldsymbol{\zeta} = (\zeta_1, \ldots, \zeta_k)^t \in \Xi^* .$$

Proof

(a) Let $\boldsymbol{Z} = (Z_1, \ldots, Z_k)^t$ and $\boldsymbol{T} = (T_1, \ldots, T_k)^t$ with $Z_j(\boldsymbol{p}) = \ln(p_j)$, $\boldsymbol{p} \in \Theta$, and $T_j(\boldsymbol{x}) = x_j$, $\boldsymbol{x} \in \mathbb{N}_0^k$, for $1 \leq j \leq k$. Moreover, let $\boldsymbol{e}_j$ denote the j-th unit vector in $\mathbb{R}^k$, $1 \leq j \leq k$. Since $\boldsymbol{T}(\boldsymbol{e}_j) - \boldsymbol{T}(\boldsymbol{0}) = \boldsymbol{e}_j$, $1 \leq j \leq k$, are linearly independent in $\mathbb{R}^k$, $T_1, \ldots, T_k$ are affinely independent by Lemma 2.22. Setting $\boldsymbol{p}^{(0)} = (\exp\{-k\}, \ldots, \exp\{-k\})^t$ and $\boldsymbol{p}^{(j)} = (p_1^{(j)}, \ldots, p_k^{(j)})^t$ with $p_i^{(j)} = \exp\{-k\}$, $i \neq j$, and $p_j^{(j)} = \exp\{-k-1\}$ for $1 \leq i, j \leq k$, we find that $\boldsymbol{Z}(\boldsymbol{p}^{(j)}) - \boldsymbol{Z}(\boldsymbol{p}^{(0)}) = -\boldsymbol{e}_j$, $1 \leq j \leq k$, are linearly independent in $\mathbb{R}^k$. Again, by Lemma 2.22, $Z_1, \ldots, Z_k$ are affinely independent. The assertion then follows from Theorem 2.23.

(b) Let $\boldsymbol{\zeta} = (\zeta_1, \ldots, \zeta_k)^t \in \mathbb{R}^k$. Then,

$$\begin{aligned}
\sum_{\boldsymbol{x} \in \mathbb{N}_0^k} \exp\left\{\sum_{j=1}^{k} \zeta_j x_j\right\} h(\boldsymbol{x}) &= \sum_{n=0}^{\infty} \sum_{\boldsymbol{x} \in \mathbb{N}_0^k : \sum_{j=1}^{k} x_j = n} \exp\left\{\sum_{j=1}^{k} \zeta_j x_j\right\} h(\boldsymbol{x}) \\
&= \sum_{n=0}^{\infty} \frac{(n + r_0 - 1)!}{(r_0 - 1)!\, n!} \sum_{\boldsymbol{x} \in \mathbb{N}_0^k : \sum_{j=1}^{k} x_j = n} \frac{n!}{\prod_{j=1}^{k} x_j!} \prod_{j=1}^{k} \left(e^{\zeta_j}\right)^{x_j} \\
&= \sum_{n=0}^{\infty} \binom{n + r_0 - 1}{r_0 - 1} \left(\sum_{j=1}^{k} e^{\zeta_j}\right)^n ,
\end{aligned}$$

where the last equation follows from the multinomial theorem. By D'Alembert's criterion, this series converges if $\sum_{j=1}^{k} \exp\{\zeta_j\} < 1$ and diverges if $\sum_{j=1}^{k} \exp\{\zeta_j\} \geq 1$. This gives Ξ^* as stated.

(c) From assertion (b), we have that $\boldsymbol{Z}(\Theta) = \Xi^*$ and Ξ^* is open, such that $\mathcal{P}$ is regular. By setting $\zeta_j = \ln(p_j)$, $1 \leq j \leq k$, in density function $f_{\boldsymbol{p}}$, the canonical representation is obtained, which is minimal according to statement (a). □

Utilizing this finding, the mean vector and covariance matrix of the negative multinomial distribution are directly obtained.

Theorem 6.3 *Let $\mathcal{P} = \mathfrak{nm}(r_0, \bullet)$ for some fixed $r_0 \in \mathbb{N}$ with minimal canonical representation (6.3). Then, the mean vector and the covariance matrix of $\boldsymbol{X} \sim P_{\boldsymbol{\zeta}}^*$ are given by*

$$\mathbb{E}_{\boldsymbol{\zeta}}(\boldsymbol{X}) = \left(\frac{r_0 e^{\zeta_1}}{1 - \sum_{j=1}^{k} e^{\zeta_j}}, \ldots, \frac{r_0 e^{\zeta_k}}{1 - \sum_{j=1}^{k} e^{\zeta_j}} \right)^t \tag{6.4}$$

and

$$\mathbb{C}\mathrm{ov}_{\boldsymbol{\zeta}}(X_i, X_j) = \frac{r_0}{1 - \sum_{l=1}^{k} e^{\zeta_l}} \left(\frac{e^{\zeta_i + \zeta_j}}{1 - \sum_{l=1}^{k} e^{\zeta_l}} + \delta_{ij}\, e^{\zeta_i} \right), \qquad 1 \leq i, j \leq k, \tag{6.5}$$

where δ_{ij} is the Kronecker delta, i.e., $\delta_{ij} = 1$ for $i = j$, and $\delta_{ij} = 0$ for $i \neq j$.

Proof Applying Corollary 2.50, we have $\mathbb{E}_{\boldsymbol{\zeta}}(\boldsymbol{X}) = E_{\boldsymbol{\zeta}}[\boldsymbol{T}] = \nabla\kappa(\boldsymbol{\zeta})$ and $\mathbb{C}\mathrm{ov}_{\boldsymbol{\zeta}}(\boldsymbol{X}) = \mathbf{Cov}_{\boldsymbol{\zeta}}(\boldsymbol{T}) = \mathbf{H}_{\kappa}(\boldsymbol{\zeta})$ for $\boldsymbol{\zeta} \in \Xi^*$, which leads to the stated formulas. □

In terms of the original parameters $p_1, \ldots, p_k$, the mean vector and covariance matrix of $\mathfrak{nm}(r_0, \boldsymbol{p})$ can be obtained by setting $\zeta_j = \ln(p_j)$, $1 \leq j \leq k$, in formulas (6.4) and (6.5).

Noticing that one-dimensional marginals are negative binomial distributions (see [28, Chapter 36]), the expressions in Theorem 6.3 for one-dimensional marginal expectations and variances are known from Example 2.51. More precisely, the parameters of the j-th marginal distribution are r_0 and $(1 - \sum_{i=1}^{n} p_i)/(1 - \sum_{i=1, i\neq j}^{n} p_i)$.

As two by-products of Theorem 6.3, the mean value function of $\mathcal{P}$ turns out to be

$$\pi(\boldsymbol{\zeta}) = \left(\frac{r_0 e^{\zeta_1}}{1 - \sum_{j=1}^{k} e^{\zeta_j}}, \ldots, \frac{r_0 e^{\zeta_k}}{1 - \sum_{j=1}^{k} e^{\zeta_j}} \right)^t, \qquad \boldsymbol{\zeta} \in \Xi^*, \tag{6.6}$$

and the Fisher information matrix of $\mathcal{P}$ at $\boldsymbol{\zeta} \in \Xi^*$ is given by

$$[\mathbf{I}(\boldsymbol{\zeta})]_{i,j} = \frac{r_0}{1-\sum_{l=1}^k e^{\zeta_l}} \left(\frac{e^{\zeta_i+\zeta_j}}{1-\sum_{l=1}^k e^{\zeta_l}} + \delta_{ij} e^{\zeta_i} \right), \qquad 1 \le i, j \le k \tag{6.7}$$

(see Theorem 2.56 and Theorem 3.29).

Let us now develop inferential results for the negative multinomial distribution. For simplicity, we restrict ourselves to the case of a single observation from $P_{\boldsymbol{\zeta}}^*$. First, maximum likelihood estimation of the natural parameters $\zeta_1, \ldots, \zeta_k$ is considered.

Theorem 6.4 *Let $\mathcal{P} = \mathfrak{nm}(r_0, \bullet)$ for some fixed $r_0 \in \mathbb{N}$ with minimal canonical representation (6.3), and let $\boldsymbol{x} \in \mathbb{N}_0^k$ be a realization of $\boldsymbol{X} \sim P_{\boldsymbol{\zeta}}^*$ for some $\boldsymbol{\zeta} \in \Xi^*$. Then, an ML estimate of $\boldsymbol{\zeta}$ in Ξ^* based on $\boldsymbol{x}$ exists if and only if $\boldsymbol{x} \in (0, \infty)^k$. If it exists, it is uniquely determined and given by*

$$\left(\ln\left(\frac{x_1}{r_0 + \sum_{i=1}^k x_i} \right), \ldots, \ln\left(\frac{x_k}{r_0 + \sum_{i=1}^k x_i} \right) \right)^t .$$

Proof From Theorem 4.3, we obtain that an ML estimate of $\boldsymbol{\zeta}$ in Ξ^* based on $\boldsymbol{x}$ exists if and only if $\boldsymbol{x} \in int(M)$, where $M = [0, \infty)^k$ is the convex support of $\boldsymbol{X}$. Hence, the first statement is clear. Now, let us compute the ML estimate $\pi^{-1}(\boldsymbol{x})$ of $\boldsymbol{\zeta}$ for $\boldsymbol{x} \in (0, \infty)^k$, where π^{-1} is the inverse function of $\pi : \Xi^* \to (0, \infty)^k$ in formula (6.6). Suppose that $\pi(\boldsymbol{\zeta}) = \boldsymbol{x}$ for some $\boldsymbol{\zeta} \in \Xi^*$. Summing up all k equations of this system then gives

$$\frac{r_0 \sum_{j=1}^k e^{\zeta_j}}{1 - \sum_{i=1}^k e^{\zeta_i}} = \sum_{j=1}^k x_j ,$$

which is equivalent to

$$\sum_{i=1}^k e^{\zeta_i} = \frac{\sum_{j=1}^k x_j}{r_0 + \sum_{j=1}^k x_j} .$$

Thus, for $1 \le j \le r$, since $r_0 \exp\{\zeta_j\}/(1 - \sum_{i=1}^k \exp\{\zeta_i\}) = x_j$, we find

$$\zeta_j = \ln\left(\frac{x_j}{r_0} \left(1 - \sum_{i=1}^k e^{\zeta_i} \right) \right) = \ln\left(\frac{x_j}{r_0 + \sum_{i=1}^k x_i} \right) .$$

□

In particular, Theorem 6.4 yields that the probability of non-existence of an ML estimate based on a single observation of $\boldsymbol{X}$ is positive, since

$$\mathbb{P}_{\boldsymbol{\zeta}}(\boldsymbol{X} \notin (0,\infty)^k) \geq \mathbb{P}_{\boldsymbol{\zeta}}(\boldsymbol{X} = \mathbf{0}) = \left(1 - \sum_{j=1}^{k} e^{\zeta_j}\right)^{r_0} > 0\,.$$

If an estimator for the mean vector of $\mathrm{nm}(r_0, \boldsymbol{p})$ is desired, then one may choose $\boldsymbol{X}$ itself.

Theorem 6.5 *Under the assumptions of Theorem 6.4, $\boldsymbol{X}$ is an efficient estimator of π, i.e., its covariance matrix attains the lower bound of the Cramér-Rao inequality given by*

$$[\mathbf{I}(\boldsymbol{\zeta})^{-1}]_{i,j} = \frac{1 - \sum_{l=1}^{k} e^{\zeta_l}}{r_0} \left(e^{-\zeta_i}\,\delta_{ij} - 1\right), \qquad 1 \leq i, j \leq k\,.$$

Proof $\boldsymbol{X}$ is an efficient estimator of π by Theorem 4.26. To find the inverse of $\mathbf{I}(\boldsymbol{\zeta})$ in formula (6.7), note that

$$\mathbf{I}(\boldsymbol{\zeta}) = \frac{r_0}{a}\left(\mathbf{P} + \frac{\boldsymbol{p}\boldsymbol{p}^t}{a}\right)$$

for the diagonal matrix $\mathbf{P}$ with positive diagonal entries $p_j = e^{\zeta_j}$, $1 \leq j \leq k$, positive number $a = 1 - \sum_{j=1}^{k} p_j$, and vector $\boldsymbol{p} = (p_1, \ldots, p_k)^t$. A well known matrix identity (see, e.g., [45, p. 458]) then yields that

$$\begin{aligned}\mathbf{I}(\boldsymbol{\zeta})^{-1} &= \frac{a}{r_0}\left(\mathbf{P}^{-1} - \mathbf{P}^{-1}\boldsymbol{p}\left(a + \boldsymbol{p}^t\mathbf{P}^{-1}\boldsymbol{p}\right)^{-1}\boldsymbol{p}^t\mathbf{P}^{-1}\right)\\ &= \frac{a}{r_0}\left(\mathbf{P}^{-1} - (1,\ldots,1)^t\,(1,\ldots,1)\right),\end{aligned}$$

noticing that $\boldsymbol{p}^t\mathbf{P}^{-1}\boldsymbol{p} = \sum_{j=1}^{k} p_j$. Inserting for $p_1, \ldots, p_k$ and a completes the proof. □

Next, suppose we are interested to statistically confirm that the probability p_1 of outcome O_1 in a single experiment exceeds a certain threshold $p_0 \in (0, 1)$, say. The corresponding test problem is

$$H_0 : p_1 \leq p_0 \qquad \leftrightarrow \qquad H_1 : p_1 > p_0 \tag{6.8}$$

or, equivalently and in terms of the natural parameter ζ_1,

$$H_0 : \zeta_1 \leq \zeta_0 \quad \leftrightarrow \quad H_1 : \zeta_1 > \zeta_0 \tag{6.9}$$

with $\zeta_0 = \ln(p_0)$. An optimal test for these test problems can be obtained from Theorem 5.12(a) by using that the conditional distribution of X_1 given $(X_2, \dots, X_k) = \boldsymbol{y}$ is a negative binomial distribution with respective parameters.

Theorem 6.6 *Let the assumptions of Theorem 6.4 be given, and let $\alpha \in (0, 1)$. Then, for test problems (6.8) and (6.9),*

$$\varphi(\boldsymbol{x}) = \mathbb{1}_{(c(\boldsymbol{y}),\infty)}(x_1) + \gamma(\boldsymbol{y})\mathbb{1}_{\{c(\boldsymbol{y})\}}(x_1), \qquad \boldsymbol{x} = (x_1, \boldsymbol{y}) \in \mathbb{N}_0^k,$$

forms a UMPU level-α test, where, for $\boldsymbol{y} = (x_2, \dots, x_k) \in \mathbb{N}_0^{k-1}$, $c(\boldsymbol{y})$ is the minimum number $m \in \mathbb{N}_0$ satisfying

$$\sum_{i=m+1}^{\infty} g_{\boldsymbol{y}}(i) \leq \alpha,$$

and

$$\gamma(\boldsymbol{y}) = \frac{\alpha - \sum_{i=c(\boldsymbol{y})+1}^{\infty} g_{\boldsymbol{y}}(i)}{g_{\boldsymbol{y}}(c(\boldsymbol{y}))},$$

where $g_{\boldsymbol{y}}$ denotes the counting density of $\mathfrak{nb}(r_0 + \sum_{i=2}^{k} x_i, 1 - e^{\zeta_0})$ defined by Example 2.5.

Let us now consider the multivariate test problem

$$H_0 : \boldsymbol{p} = \boldsymbol{q} \quad \leftrightarrow \quad H_1 : \boldsymbol{p} \neq \boldsymbol{q} \tag{6.10}$$

with a simple null hypothesis and fixed $\boldsymbol{q} = (q_1, \dots, q_k)^t \in \Theta$, or, equivalently and in terms of the natural parameter $\boldsymbol{\zeta}$,

$$H_0 : \boldsymbol{\zeta} = \boldsymbol{\eta} \quad \leftrightarrow \quad H_1 : \boldsymbol{\zeta} \neq \boldsymbol{\eta} \tag{6.11}$$

with $\boldsymbol{\eta} = (\eta_1, \dots, \eta_k)^t \in \Xi^*$ defined by $\eta_j = \ln(q_j)$, $1 \leq j \leq k$. Since the MLE of $\boldsymbol{\zeta}$ in Ξ^* based on $\boldsymbol{X}$ does not exist a.s., we focus on the Rao score test, which, in contrast to the LR test and the Wald test, does not depend on the MLE in Ξ^*.

Theorem 6.7 *Under the assumptions of Theorem 6.4, the test statistic of the Rao score test for test problems (6.10) and (6.11) is given by*

$$R(\boldsymbol{x}) = \frac{1 - \sum_{i=1}^{k} e^{\eta_i}}{r_0} \left\{ \sum_{j=1}^{k} e^{-\eta_j} \left(x_j - \frac{r_0 e^{\eta_j}}{1 - \sum_{i=1}^{k} e^{\eta_i}} \right)^2 - \left[\sum_{j=1}^{k} \left(x_j - \frac{r_0 e^{\eta_j}}{1 - \sum_{i=1}^{k} e^{\eta_i}} \right) \right]^2 \right\}$$

for $\boldsymbol{x} = (x_1, \ldots, x_k)^t \in \mathbb{N}_0^k$.

Proof By using the same notation as in the proof of Theorem 6.5, we have

$$\boldsymbol{U}_{\boldsymbol{\zeta}}^t \, \mathbf{I}(\boldsymbol{\zeta})^{-1} \, \boldsymbol{U}_{\boldsymbol{\zeta}} = \frac{a}{r_0} \left\{ \boldsymbol{U}_{\boldsymbol{\zeta}}^t \, \mathbf{P}^{-1} \, \boldsymbol{U}_{\boldsymbol{\zeta}} - \left[(1, \ldots, 1) \, \boldsymbol{U}_{\boldsymbol{\zeta}} \right]^2 \right\}$$

Moreover, we conclude from Theorem 3.29 together with formula (6.4) that the score statistic at $\boldsymbol{\zeta}$ is given by $\boldsymbol{U}_{\boldsymbol{\zeta}}(\boldsymbol{x}) = \boldsymbol{x} - r_0 \boldsymbol{p}/a$, $\boldsymbol{x} \in \mathbb{N}_0^k$. Inserting for $a, p_1, \ldots, p_k$, and replacing $\boldsymbol{\zeta}$ by $\boldsymbol{\eta}$ then gives the representation for R defined in Remark 5.17. □

The Rao score test then rejects the null hypothesis if R in Theorem 6.7 exceeds a certain critical value. Since $\boldsymbol{X}$ is discrete so is R, and to guarantee that the test has exact level $\alpha \in (0, 1)$ therefore requires a randomized test based on R, in general. A non-randomized level-α test, which rejects H_0 if and only if R exceeds the critical value, can be obtained if the critical value is determined as the $(1 - \alpha)$-quantile $r_{1-\alpha}$, say, of R under H_0, i.e., if $\boldsymbol{\zeta} = \boldsymbol{\eta}$ is true. By doing so, the exact level of the test may be smaller than α, in the case of which the test is also called *conservative*. To compute a numerical value for $r_{1-\alpha}$, Monte-Carlo simulation can be used, where a sufficiently large number of realizations of R are generated under the assumption that $\boldsymbol{\zeta} = \boldsymbol{\eta}$, and then the empirical $(1 - \alpha)$-quantile of the resulting data vector is chosen for $r_{1-\alpha}$. Here, note that the convergence of the empirical $(1 - \alpha)$-quantile to the true $(1 - \alpha)$-quantile for increasing simulation size is only guaranteed if the quantile function of R is continuous at $1 - \alpha$ (see, e.g., [58, pp. 304/305]).

Finally, inverting the acceptance region of the test also yields a confidence region for $\boldsymbol{\zeta}$, i.e.,

$$C(\boldsymbol{x}) = \{\boldsymbol{\zeta} \in \Xi^* : R(\boldsymbol{x}) \leq r_{1-\alpha}\}, \qquad \boldsymbol{x} \in \mathcal{X},$$

with (at least) level $1 - \alpha$. A confidence region for the original parameter $\boldsymbol{p}$ with (at least) level $1 - \alpha$ is then given by

$$\tilde{C}(\boldsymbol{x}) = \left\{ \left(e^{\zeta_1}, \ldots, e^{\zeta_k}\right)^t : (\zeta_1, \ldots, \zeta_k)^t \in C(\boldsymbol{x}) \right\}, \qquad \boldsymbol{x} \in \mathcal{X}.$$

6.2 Dirichlet Distribution

The Dirichlet distribution is a multivariate extension of the beta distribution, and it is widely used in the literature (see, e.g., [37, Chapter 49] and [47]).

Definition 6.8 The *Dirichlet distribution* $\mathcal{D}(\boldsymbol{\beta})$ with parameter vector $\boldsymbol{\beta} = (\beta_1, \ldots, \beta_{k+1})^t \in (0, \infty)^{k+1}$, $k \in \mathbb{N}$, is defined as the distribution on the Borel sets of $\mathcal{X} = \{(y_1, \ldots, y_k)^t \in (0,1)^k : \sum_{i=1}^k y_i < 1\}$ with Lebesgue density function

$$f_{\boldsymbol{\beta}}(\boldsymbol{x}) = \frac{1}{B(\boldsymbol{\beta})} \left(\prod_{j=1}^{k} x_j^{\beta_j - 1} \right) \left(1 - \sum_{j=1}^{k} x_j \right)^{\beta_{k+1}-1} \tag{6.12}$$

for $\boldsymbol{x} = (x_1, \ldots, x_k)^t \in \mathcal{X}$, where B denotes the beta function, i.e.,

$$B(\boldsymbol{\beta}) = \frac{\prod_{i=1}^{k+1} \Gamma(\beta_i)}{\Gamma(\sum_{i=1}^{k+1} \beta_i)}, \qquad \boldsymbol{\beta} \in (0, \infty)^{k+1}. \tag{6.13}$$

By setting $k = 1$ in Definition 6.8, $\mathcal{D}(\beta_1, \beta_2)$ coincides with the beta distribution $\mathcal{B}(\beta_1, \beta_2)$, $\beta_1, \beta_2 \in (0, \infty)$.

According to Example 2.13, we may rewrite density function (6.12) as

$$f_{\boldsymbol{\beta}}(\boldsymbol{x}) = \frac{1}{B(\boldsymbol{\beta})} \exp\left\{ \sum_{j=1}^{k+1} \beta_j T_j(\boldsymbol{x}) \right\} h(\boldsymbol{x}) \tag{6.14}$$

with statistics

$$T_j(\boldsymbol{x}) = \ln(x_j), \quad 1 \le j \le k, \qquad T_{k+1}(\boldsymbol{x}) = \ln\left(1 - \sum_{i=1}^{k} x_i\right), \tag{6.15}$$

and function

$$h(\boldsymbol{x}) = \left[\left(1 - \sum_{j=1}^{k} x_j \right) \prod_{j=1}^{k} x_j \right]^{-1} \tag{6.16}$$

for $\boldsymbol{x} \in \mathcal{X}$. Hence, $\mathcal{P} = \mathcal{D}(\bullet) = \{\mathcal{D}(\boldsymbol{\beta}) : \boldsymbol{\beta} \in (0,\infty)^{k+1}\}$ forms an EF. Note that formula (6.14) is already a canonical representation of $\mathcal{P}$.

Some properties of $\mathcal{D}(\bullet)$ are stated in the following theorem, where the proof of assertion (a) is technical and therefore omitted.

Theorem 6.9 *For $\mathcal{P} = \mathcal{D}(\bullet)$ as introduced above, we find:*

(a) $ord(\mathcal{P}) = k+1$.
(b) The natural parameter space of $\mathcal{P}$ is given by $\Xi^* = (0,\infty)^{k+1}$.
(c) $\mathcal{P}$ is regular with minimal canonical representation given by the Lebesgue density functions

$$f_{\boldsymbol{\beta}}(\boldsymbol{x}) = \frac{dP_{\boldsymbol{\beta}}}{d\lambda_{\mathcal{X}}}(\boldsymbol{x}) = e^{\boldsymbol{\beta}^t \boldsymbol{T}(\boldsymbol{x}) - \kappa(\boldsymbol{\beta})}\, h(\boldsymbol{x}), \qquad \boldsymbol{x} \in \mathcal{X}, \tag{6.17}$$

for $\boldsymbol{\beta} \in (0,\infty)^{k+1}$, where $\boldsymbol{T} = (T_1,\ldots,T_{k+1})^t$ with T_j, $1 \le j \le k+1$, as in formula (6.15), h as in formula (6.16), and cumulant function $\kappa = \ln(B)$ on $(0,\infty)^{k+1}$ with B as in formula (6.13).

Proof

(b) Evidently, we have $(0,\infty)^{k+1} \subset \Xi^*$. Let $\beta_2,\ldots,\beta_{k+1} \in [0,\infty)$ and note that $h(\boldsymbol{x}) \ge 1/x_1$ for $\boldsymbol{x} \in \mathcal{X}$. By introducing the k-dimensional rectangle $\mathcal{Y} = I \times J^{k-1} \subset \mathcal{X}$ with $I = (0, 1/(k+1))$ and $J = (1/(k+2), 1/(k+1))$, we have for $\boldsymbol{x} \in \mathcal{Y}$ that

$$\begin{aligned}\exp\left\{\sum_{j=2}^{k+1} \beta_j T_j(\boldsymbol{x})\right\} h(\boldsymbol{x}) &\ge \left(\prod_{j=2}^{k} x_j^{\beta_j}\right)\left(1 - \sum_{j=1}^{k} x_j\right)^{\beta_{k+1}} \frac{1}{x_1}\\ &\ge \left(\prod_{j=2}^{k}\left(\frac{1}{k+2}\right)^{\beta_j}\right)\left(1 - \frac{k}{k+1}\right)^{\beta_{k+1}} \frac{1}{x_1} = \frac{d}{x_1},\end{aligned}$$

say, where $d > 0$. Hence,

$$\begin{aligned}\int_{\mathcal{X}} \exp\left\{\sum_{j=2}^{k+1} \beta_j T_j\right\} h\, d\lambda_{\mathcal{X}} &\ge \int_{\mathcal{Y}} \exp\left\{\sum_{j=2}^{k+1} \beta_j T_j\right\} h\, d\lambda_{\mathcal{X}} \ge d \int_{\mathcal{Y}} \frac{1}{x_1}\, d\lambda_{\mathcal{X}}(\boldsymbol{x})\\ &= d\left(\frac{1}{k+1} - \frac{1}{k+2}\right)^{k-1} \int_0^{1/(k+1)} \frac{1}{x_1}\, dx_1 = \infty.\end{aligned}$$

Hence, $(0,\beta_2,\ldots,\beta_{k+1})^t \notin \Xi^*$ for $\beta_2,\ldots,\beta_{k+1} \in [0,\infty)$. For symmetry reasons, we even have that $(\beta_1,\ldots,\beta_{k+1})^t \notin \Xi^*$ for $\beta_i \in [0,\infty)$, $1 \le i \le k+1$, if $\beta_j = 0$ for some $j \in \{1, \ldots, k+1\}$. Since Ξ^* is convex by Theorem 2.34, it follows that $\Xi^* = (0, \infty)^{k+1}$.

(c) The assertion follows directly from (a) and (b). □

The mean vector and the covariance matrix of $\boldsymbol{T}$ are now readily derived.

Theorem 6.10 *Let $\mathcal{P} = \mathcal{D}(\bullet)$ with minimal canonical representation (6.17). Then, the mean vector and the covariance matrix of $\boldsymbol{T}$ under $P_{\boldsymbol{\beta}}$ are given by*

$$E_{\boldsymbol{\beta}}(\boldsymbol{T}) = \left(\psi(\beta_1) - \psi(\boldsymbol{\beta}_\bullet), \ldots, \psi(\beta_{k+1}) - \psi(\boldsymbol{\beta}_\bullet)\right)^t$$

and

$$Cov_{\boldsymbol{\beta}}(T_i, T_j) = \psi'(\beta_i)\,\delta_{ij} - \psi'(\boldsymbol{\beta}_\bullet), \qquad 1 \le i, j \le k+1,$$

where $\psi = [\ln(\Gamma)]' = \Gamma'/\Gamma$ denotes the digamma function, δ_{ij} is the Kronecker delta, i.e., $\delta_{ij} = 1$ for $i = j$, and $\delta_{ij} = 0$ for $i \neq j$, and the notation $\boldsymbol{\beta}_\bullet = \sum_{i=1}^{k+1} \beta_i$ is used for $\boldsymbol{\beta} \in (0, \infty)^{k+1}$.

Proof Applying Corollary 2.50, we have for $1 \le j \le k+1$ that $E_{\boldsymbol{\beta}}(T_j) = \partial/\partial\beta_j\, \kappa(\boldsymbol{\beta}) = [\partial/\partial\beta_j\, B(\boldsymbol{\beta})]/B(\boldsymbol{\beta})$ and $\mathbf{Cov}_{\boldsymbol{\beta}}(\boldsymbol{T}) = \mathbf{H}_\kappa(\boldsymbol{\beta})$, from which the assertions follow by elementary calculus. □

As two by-products of Theorem 6.10, the mean value function of $\mathcal{P}$ turns out to be

$$\pi(\boldsymbol{\beta}) = \left(\psi(\beta_1) - \psi(\boldsymbol{\beta}_\bullet), \ldots, \psi(\beta_{k+1}) - \psi(\boldsymbol{\beta}_\bullet)\right)^t, \qquad \boldsymbol{\beta} \in (0, \infty)^{k+1}, \tag{6.18}$$

and the Fisher information matrix of $\mathcal{P}$ at $\boldsymbol{\beta} \in (0, \infty)^{k+1}$ is given by

$$[\mathbf{I}(\boldsymbol{\beta})]_{i,j} = \psi'(\beta_i)\,\delta_{ij} - \psi'(\boldsymbol{\beta}_\bullet), \qquad 1 \le i, j \le k+1 \tag{6.19}$$

(see Theorems 2.56 and 3.29).

Now, we turn to inferential results for the Dirichlet distribution based on an iid sample from $P_{\boldsymbol{\beta}}$. We start with maximum likelihood estimation of the natural parameters $\beta_1, \ldots, \beta_{k+1}$. To apply the results of Sect. 4.1, note first that the boundary of the convex support of $\boldsymbol{T}$ is nothing but the support $\{\boldsymbol{T}(\boldsymbol{x}) : \boldsymbol{x} \in \mathcal{X}\}$ of $\boldsymbol{T}$, i.e.,

$$\partial M = \left\{ \left(\ln(x_1), \ldots, \ln(x_k), \ln\left(1 - \sum_{j=1}^{k} x_j\right)\right)^t : \boldsymbol{x} \in (0,1)^k,\ \sum_{j=1}^{k} x_j < 1 \right\} \tag{6.20}$$

Theorem 4.3 then yields that an ML estimate based on a single observation $\boldsymbol{x}$ from $P_{\boldsymbol{\beta}}$ does not exist, since $\boldsymbol{T}(\boldsymbol{x}) \in \partial M$ $P_{\boldsymbol{\beta}}$-a.s.. However, for a sample size larger than 1, we have the following theorem (see also [20, pp. 150–152] for the particular case of the beta distribution).

Theorem 6.11 *Let $\mathcal{P} = \mathcal{D}(\bullet)$ with minimal canonical representation (6.17), and let $\boldsymbol{x}^{(1)}, \ldots, \boldsymbol{x}^{(n)} \in \mathcal{X}$ be realizations of iid random vectors $\boldsymbol{X}^{(1)}, \ldots, \boldsymbol{X}^{(n)}$ with distribution $P_{\boldsymbol{\beta}}$ for some $\boldsymbol{\beta} \in (0, \infty)^{k+1}$. If $n \geq 2$ and $\boldsymbol{x}^{(1)}, \ldots, \boldsymbol{x}^{(n)}$ are not all identical, then an ML estimate of $\boldsymbol{\beta}$ in $(0, \infty)^{k+1}$ based on $\boldsymbol{x}^{(1)}, \ldots, \boldsymbol{x}^{(n)}$ uniquely exists and is given by the only solution of the equations*

$$\psi(\beta_j) - \psi(\boldsymbol{\beta}_\bullet) = \frac{1}{n}\sum_{i=1}^{n} \ln(x_j^{(i)}), \qquad 1 \leq j \leq k,$$

$$\text{and} \qquad \psi(\beta_{k+1}) - \psi(\boldsymbol{\beta}_\bullet) = \frac{1}{n}\sum_{i=1}^{n} \ln\left(1 - \sum_{l=1}^{k} x_l^{(i)}\right)$$

with respect to $\boldsymbol{\beta} \in (0, \infty)^{k+1}$. Moreover, the MLE $\hat{\boldsymbol{\beta}}^{(n)}$ of $\boldsymbol{\beta}$ in $(0, \infty)^{k+1}$ based on $\boldsymbol{X}^{(1)}, \ldots, \boldsymbol{X}^{(n)}$ uniquely exists (a.s.) for all $n \geq 2$.

Proof Let $\boldsymbol{x}^{(1)}, \ldots, \boldsymbol{x}^{(n)} \in \mathcal{X}$ with $\boldsymbol{x}^{(i)} = (x_1^{(i)}, \ldots, x_k^{(i)})^t$, $1 \leq i \leq n$, be not all identical. By Corollary 4.5 and Remark 4.4, we have to show that

$$\frac{1}{n}\sum_{i=1}^{n} \boldsymbol{T}(\boldsymbol{x}^{(i)}) \notin \partial M,$$

where ∂M is given by formula (6.20). For this, suppose that there exists some $\boldsymbol{y} = (y_1, \ldots, y_k)^t \in \mathcal{X}$ with

$$\begin{aligned} \frac{1}{n}\sum_{i=1}^{n} T_j(\boldsymbol{x}^{(i)}) &= \frac{1}{n}\sum_{i=1}^{n} \ln(x_j^{(i)}) \\ &= \ln(y_j), \qquad 1 \leq j \leq k. \end{aligned}$$

Then, two-fold application of the inequality of arithmetic and geometric mean yields that

$$\begin{aligned} \frac{1}{n}\sum_{i=1}^{n} T_{k+1}(\boldsymbol{x}^{(i)}) &= \frac{1}{n}\sum_{i=1}^{n} \ln\left(1 - \sum_{j=1}^{k} x_j^{(i)}\right) = \ln\left(\left[\prod_{i=1}^{n}\left(1 - \sum_{j=1}^{k} x_j^{(i)}\right)\right]^{1/n}\right) \\ &\leq \ln\left(\frac{1}{n}\sum_{i=1}^{n}\left[1 - \sum_{j=1}^{k} x_j^{(i)}\right]\right) = \ln\left(1 - \sum_{j=1}^{k}\frac{1}{n}\sum_{i=1}^{n} x_j^{(i)}\right) \\ &< \ln\left(1 - \sum_{j=1}^{k}\left[\prod_{i=1}^{n} x_j^{(i)}\right]^{1/n}\right) = \ln\left(1 - \sum_{j=1}^{k} y_j\right), \end{aligned}$$

i.e., $\sum_{i=1}^{n} \boldsymbol{T}(\boldsymbol{x}^{(i)})/n \notin \partial M$, and an ML estimate of $\boldsymbol{\beta}$ based on $\boldsymbol{x}^{(1)}, \ldots, \boldsymbol{x}^{(n)}$ uniquely exists. Since $\boldsymbol{x}^{(1)} = \cdots = \boldsymbol{x}^{(n)}$ occurs with $P_{\boldsymbol{\beta}}$-probability 0, the proof is done. □

For $n \geq 2$, the MLE $\hat{\boldsymbol{\beta}}^{(n)}$ of $\boldsymbol{\beta}$ in Theorem 6.11 cannot be stated explicitly, and an ML estimate based on (non-identical) realizations $\boldsymbol{x}^{(1)}, \ldots, \boldsymbol{x}^{(n)}$ has to be obtained via numerical procedures (see [37, pp. 505/506] and also [27, pp. 223–225] in case of the beta distribution). In contrast, we have the explicit MLE $\sum_{i=1}^{n} \boldsymbol{T}(\boldsymbol{X}^{(i)})/n$ of $\pi(\boldsymbol{\beta})$ based on $\boldsymbol{X}^{(1)}, \ldots, \boldsymbol{X}^{(n)}$, which is moreover efficient by Corollary 4.27.

Since the MLE of the natural parameter $\boldsymbol{\beta}$ is not available in explicit form, we cannot derive its exact distribution analytically, which however is required, e.g., for the construction of statistical tests and confidence regions for $\boldsymbol{\beta}$. We therefore now assume to have a sequence of iid random vectors following a Dirichlet distribution and focus on asymptotic inferential results.

Theorem 6.12 *Let $\mathcal{P} = \mathcal{D}(\bullet)$ with minimal canonical representation (6.17), and let $\boldsymbol{X}^{(1)}, \boldsymbol{X}^{(2)}, \ldots$ be a sequence of iid random vectors with distribution $P_{\boldsymbol{\beta}}$ for some $\boldsymbol{\beta} \in (0, \infty)^{k+1}$. Then, the sequence $\hat{\boldsymbol{\beta}}^{(n)}$, $n \in \mathbb{N}$, $n \geq 2$, of MLEs for $\boldsymbol{\beta}$ is strongly consistent and asymptotically efficient for $\boldsymbol{\beta}$, i.e., we have $\hat{\boldsymbol{\beta}}^{(n)} \to \boldsymbol{\beta}$ $\mathbb{P}_{\boldsymbol{\beta}}$-a.s. and*

$$\sqrt{n}(\hat{\boldsymbol{\beta}}^{(n)} - \boldsymbol{\beta}) \xrightarrow{d} \mathcal{N}_{k+1}(\mathbf{0}, \mathbf{I}(\boldsymbol{\beta})^{-1})$$

for $n \to \infty$, where the inverse of the Fisher information matrix at $\boldsymbol{\beta}$ is given by

$$[\mathbf{I}(\boldsymbol{\beta})^{-1}]_{i,j} = \frac{\delta_{ij}}{\psi'(\beta_i)} - \left(\sum_{l=1}^{k+1} \frac{1}{\psi'(\beta_l)} - \frac{1}{\psi'(\beta_\bullet)}\right)^{-1} \frac{1}{\psi'(\beta_i)\,\psi'(\beta_j)}$$

for $1 \leq i, j \leq k+1$.

Proof Strong consistency and asymptotic efficiency of the sequence $\hat{\boldsymbol{\beta}}^{(n)}$, $n \geq 2$, are obtained from Theorems 4.31, 4.34, and Remark 4.35. To obtain the inverse of $\mathbf{I}(\boldsymbol{\beta})$ given by formula (6.19), note that $\mathbf{I}(\boldsymbol{\beta}) = \mathbf{D} + b\boldsymbol{v}\boldsymbol{v}^t$ for the diagonal matrix $\mathbf{D}$ with diagonal entries $d_j = \psi'(\beta_j) > 0$, $1 \leq j \leq k+1$, real number $b = -\psi'(\beta_\bullet) < 0$, and vector $\boldsymbol{v} = (1, \ldots, 1)^t \in \mathbb{R}^{k+1}$. Applying a commonly known matrix identity (see, e.g., [45, p. 458]) and setting $\boldsymbol{w} = (1/d_1, \ldots, 1/d_{k+1})^t$ then yields

$$\begin{aligned}(\mathbf{D} + b\boldsymbol{v}\boldsymbol{v}^t)^{-1} &= \mathbf{D}^{-1} - \mathbf{D}^{-1}\boldsymbol{v}\left(\frac{1}{b} + \boldsymbol{v}^t\mathbf{D}^{-1}\boldsymbol{v}\right)^{-1} \boldsymbol{v}^t\mathbf{D}^{-1} \\ &= \mathbf{D}^{-1} - \left(\frac{1}{b} + \sum_{l=1}^{k+1} \frac{1}{d_l}\right)^{-1} \boldsymbol{w}\boldsymbol{w}^t .\end{aligned}$$

Inserting for $d_1, \ldots, d_{k+1}$ and b then gives the representation. □

Now, let us consider the multivariate test problem

$$H_0 : \boldsymbol{\beta} = \boldsymbol{\eta} \qquad \leftrightarrow \qquad H_1 : \boldsymbol{\beta} \neq \boldsymbol{\eta} \tag{6.21}$$

for some fixed $\boldsymbol{\eta} = (\eta_1, \ldots, \eta_{k+1})^t \in (0, \infty)^{k+1}$.

Theorem 6.13 *Under the assumptions of Theorem 6.12, the test statistics $\Lambda_n = \Lambda_n(\boldsymbol{X}^{(1)}, \ldots, \boldsymbol{X}^{(n)})$ and $W_n = W_n(\boldsymbol{X}^{(1)}, \ldots, \boldsymbol{X}^{(n)})$ of the LR test and the Wald test (with $g(\boldsymbol{\beta}) = \boldsymbol{\beta} - \boldsymbol{\eta}$, $\boldsymbol{\beta} \in (0, \infty)^{k+1}$) for test problem (6.21) based on $\boldsymbol{X}^{(1)}, \ldots, \boldsymbol{X}^{(n)}$, $n \geq 2$, are given by*

$$\Lambda_n = 2n \left[\ln\left(\frac{B(\boldsymbol{\eta})}{B(\hat{\boldsymbol{\beta}}^{(n)})} \right) + \sum_{j=1}^{k+1} (\hat{\beta}_j^{(n)} - \eta_j) \left(\psi\left(\hat{\beta}_j^{(n)}\right) - \psi\left(\hat{\boldsymbol{\beta}}_{\bullet}^{(n)}\right) \right) \right]$$

and

$$W_n = n \left[\sum_{j=1}^{k+1} \psi'(\hat{\beta}_j^{(n)}) \left(\hat{\beta}_j^{(n)} - \eta_j\right)^2 - \psi'\left(\hat{\boldsymbol{\beta}}_{\bullet}^{(n)}\right) \left(\hat{\boldsymbol{\beta}}_{\bullet}^{(n)} - \boldsymbol{\eta}_{\bullet}\right)^2 \right].$$

Under H_0, both test statistics are asymptotically $\chi^2(k+1)$-distributed for $n \to \infty$.

Proof From Theorem 5.19 and Remark 5.21, Λ_n and W_n both have an asymptotic $\chi^2(k+1)$-distribution if H_0 is true, such that we only have to verify the representations of the test statistics. From Theorem 5.16 and Lemma 3.37, we obtain that

$$\begin{aligned} \Lambda_n &= 2n\, D_{KL}(\hat{\boldsymbol{\beta}}^{(n)}, \boldsymbol{\eta}) \\ &= 2n \left[\kappa(\boldsymbol{\eta}) - \kappa(\hat{\boldsymbol{\beta}}^{(n)}) + (\hat{\boldsymbol{\beta}}^{(n)} - \boldsymbol{\eta})^t \pi(\hat{\boldsymbol{\beta}}^{(n)}) \right], \end{aligned}$$

and the representation follows from $\kappa = \ln(B)$ and formula (6.18). Here, note that nD_{KL} is the Kullback-Leibler divergence corresponding to the product family $\mathcal{P}^{(n)}$.

To obtain the formula for W_n as introduced in Remark 5.17 note first that by Theorem 3.29 the Fisher information matrix at $\boldsymbol{\beta}$ for the product family $\mathcal{P}^{(n)}$ is given by $n\mathbf{I}(\boldsymbol{\beta})$. Hence, by using the same notation as in the proof of Theorem 6.12, we find

$$(\boldsymbol{\beta} - \boldsymbol{\eta})^t \, [n\,\mathbf{I}(\boldsymbol{\beta})]\, (\boldsymbol{\beta} - \boldsymbol{\eta}) = n \left\{ (\boldsymbol{\beta} - \boldsymbol{\eta})^t \,\mathbf{D}\, (\boldsymbol{\beta} - \boldsymbol{\eta}) + b\,[(\boldsymbol{\beta} - \boldsymbol{\eta})^t \boldsymbol{v}]^2 \right\}. \tag{6.22}$$

Inserting for $d_1, \ldots, d_{k+1}$ and b and finally setting $\boldsymbol{\beta} = \hat{\boldsymbol{\beta}}$ in formula (6.22) leads to the representation for W_n. □

For $\alpha \in (0, 1)$, the LR test and the Wald test with asymptotic level α then reject null hypothesis (6.21) if and only if the respective test statistic exceeds the critical value $\chi^2_{1-\alpha}(k+1)$, i.e., the $(1-\alpha)$-quantile of $\chi^2(k+1)$. For fixed $n \in \mathbb{N}$, the actual level of every test can be obtained by Monte-Carlo simulation. Here, a sufficiently large number of realizations of the test statistic under H_0, i.e., under the assumption that $\boldsymbol{\beta} = \boldsymbol{\eta}$ is true, are generated. The actual level of the test is then estimated by the relative frequency of exceeding $\chi^2_{1-\alpha}(k+1)$, i.e., of (falsely) rejecting H_0.

Since the above tests are non-randomized, they may also serve to construct confidence regions for $\boldsymbol{\beta}$, which asymptotically meet a desired confidence level. For instance, in case of the LR test,

$$C_{\Lambda_n}(\tilde{\boldsymbol{x}}) = \left\{\boldsymbol{\beta} \in (0,\infty)^{k+1} : \Lambda_n(\tilde{\boldsymbol{x}}) \leq \chi^2_{1-\alpha}(k+1)\right\}, \qquad \tilde{\boldsymbol{x}} \in \mathcal{X}^n,$$

forms a confidence region for $\boldsymbol{\beta}$ with asymptotic level $1-\alpha$ (for $n \to \infty$).

6.3 Generalized Order Statistics

Generalized order statistics have been introduced as a general semi-parametric model for ordered random variables, which contains, for instance, common order statistics, record values and k-record values, sequential order statistics, Pfeifer record values, and progressively type-II censored order statistics (see [31, 32]). What is remarkable here is the fact that joint density functions of generalized order statistics with a fixed but arbitrarily chosen absolutely continuous baseline distribution function F (see formula (6.23)) lead to a multiparameter EF, the support of which is a cone of $\mathbb{R}^n$.

Definition 6.14 Let F denote a distribution function with Lebesgue density function f and quantile function F^{-1}, and let $\gamma_1, \ldots, \gamma_n$ be positive parameters. Then, the random variables $X_1, \ldots, X_n$ are called *generalized order statistics* based on F and $\gamma_1, \ldots, \gamma_n$ if their joint density function is given by

$$g_{F,\boldsymbol{\gamma}}(\boldsymbol{x}) = \left(\prod_{j=1}^{n} \gamma_j\right)\left(\prod_{j=1}^{n-1}(1-F(x_j))^{\gamma_j-\gamma_{j+1}-1} f(x_j)\right)(1-F(x_n))^{\gamma_n-1} f(x_n) \tag{6.23}$$

for $\boldsymbol{x} \in \mathcal{X} = \{(x_1,\ldots,x_n)^t \in \mathbb{R}^n : F^{-1}(0+) < x_1 < \cdots < x_n < F^{-1}(1)\}$.

For $\gamma_j = n-j+1$, $1 \leq j \leq n$, formula (6.23) is the joint density function of n common order statistics based on F, and setting $\gamma_j = 1$, $1 \leq j \leq n$, yields the joint density function of n record values based on F.

In the context of sequential order statistics and Pfeifer record values, the parameters $\gamma_1, \ldots, \gamma_n$ and/or the distribution function F are typically unknown and have to be estimated based on data (see, e.g., [21, 32, 10, 11, 46]). In [8], it has been shown that formula (6.23) can be rewritten as

$$g_{F,\boldsymbol{\gamma}}(\boldsymbol{x}) = C(\boldsymbol{\gamma})\, e^{\boldsymbol{\gamma}^t \boldsymbol{T}(\boldsymbol{x})}\, h(\boldsymbol{x}), \qquad \boldsymbol{x} \in \mathcal{X},$$

where

$$C(\boldsymbol{\gamma}) = \prod_{j=1}^{n} \gamma_j\,, \qquad \boldsymbol{\gamma} = (\gamma_1, \ldots, \gamma_n)^t \in \Xi^* = (0,\infty)^n\,,$$

vector $\boldsymbol{T} = (T_1, \ldots, T_n)^t$ of statistics is defined by

$$T_j(\boldsymbol{x}) = \ln\left(\frac{1 - F(x_j)}{1 - F(x_{j-1})}\right), \qquad \boldsymbol{x} = (x_1, \ldots, x_n)^t \in \mathcal{X}\,, \qquad 1 \le j \le n\,,$$

with $F(x_0) = 0$, and the function h is given by $h(\boldsymbol{x}) = \prod_{j=1}^{n} f(x_j)/(1 - F(x_j))$ on $\mathcal{X}$. Hence, for fixed distribution function F,

$$\mathcal{P} = \{g_{F,\boldsymbol{\gamma}} \lambda_{\mathcal{X}} : \boldsymbol{\gamma} \in \Xi^*\}$$

forms an EF, which can be proven to be regular and of order n (see [8]). These findings are helpful to establish inferential properties for generalized order statistics.

First, by Lemma 3.1(a), the moment generating function of $-\boldsymbol{T}$ turns out to be

$$m_{-\boldsymbol{T}}(\boldsymbol{a}) = m_{\boldsymbol{T}}(-\boldsymbol{a}) = \frac{C(\boldsymbol{\gamma})}{C(\boldsymbol{\gamma} - \boldsymbol{a})} = \prod_{j=1}^{n} \frac{\gamma_j}{\gamma_j - a_j}$$

for $\boldsymbol{a} = (a_1, \ldots, a_n)^t \in \mathbb{R}^n$ with $a_j < \gamma_j$, $1 \le j \le n$. Since the mapping $t \mapsto \lambda/(\lambda - t)$, $t < \lambda$, is the moment generating function of the exponential distribution $\mathcal{E}(1/\lambda)$ with scale parameter $1/\lambda$, we obtain from the one-to-one correspondence of distribution and moment generating function that $T_1, \ldots, T_n$ are independent and $-T_j \sim \mathcal{E}(1/\gamma_j)$ for $1 \le j \le n$. Moments of $\boldsymbol{T}$ are therefore at hand; in particular, the mean value function is given by

$$\pi(\boldsymbol{\gamma}) = E_{\boldsymbol{\gamma}}[\boldsymbol{T}] = -(1/\gamma_1, \ldots, 1/\gamma_n)^t\,, \qquad \boldsymbol{\gamma} = (\gamma_1, \ldots, \gamma_n)^t \in \Xi^*\,,$$

and the Fisher information matrix $\mathbf{I}(\boldsymbol{\gamma})$ at $\boldsymbol{\gamma} \in \Xi^*$ is a diagonal matrix with diagonal elements $1/\gamma_j^2$, $1 \le j \le n$ (see Theorems 2.56 and 3.29).

Now, let an iid sample $\boldsymbol{X}^{(1)}, \ldots, \boldsymbol{X}^{(s)}$ from the distribution with density function $g_{F,\boldsymbol{\gamma}}$ be given, and let $\tilde{\boldsymbol{X}} = (\boldsymbol{X}^{(1)}, \ldots, \boldsymbol{X}^{(s)})$. Then, applying Theorem 3.13(b), Corollaries 3.17 and 3.21 to the product EF $\mathcal{P}^{(s)}$ yields that $\boldsymbol{T}^{(s)} = (T_1^{(s)}, \ldots, T_n^{(s)})^t$ with

$$T_j^{(s)}(\tilde{\boldsymbol{x}}) = \sum_{i=1}^{s} T_j(\boldsymbol{x}^{(i)})\,, \qquad \tilde{\boldsymbol{x}} = (\boldsymbol{x}^{(1)}, \ldots, \boldsymbol{x}^{(s)}) \in \mathcal{X}^s\,,$$

is a minimal sufficient and complete statistic for $\boldsymbol{\gamma}$. Evidently, $T_1^{(s)}, \ldots, T_n^{(s)}$ are independent with $-T_j \sim \mathcal{G}(1/\gamma_j, s)$, $1 \leq j \leq n$. By Corollary 4.5 with $\pi(\Xi^*) = (-\infty, 0)^n$, the MLE $\hat{\boldsymbol{\gamma}}^{(s)}$ of $\boldsymbol{\gamma}$ in Ξ^* based on $\tilde{\boldsymbol{X}}$ uniquely exists and is obtained as

$$\hat{\boldsymbol{\gamma}}^{(s)} = \pi^{-1}\left(\frac{1}{s}\boldsymbol{T}^{(s)}(\tilde{\boldsymbol{X}})\right) = -\left(s/T_1^{(s)}(\tilde{\boldsymbol{X}}), \ldots, s/T_n^{(s)}(\tilde{\boldsymbol{X}})\right)^t$$

with independent components, which are inverse gamma-distributed (since the statistics $T_1^{(s)}, \ldots, T_n^{(s)}$ are independent and gamma-distributed). According to Corollary 4.27, the vector of the reciprocals of $\gamma_1, \ldots, \gamma_n$ can efficiently be estimated by $-\boldsymbol{T}^{(s)}(\tilde{\boldsymbol{X}})/s$. Moreover, Theorems 4.31 and 4.34 guarantee strong consistency and asymptotic efficiency of the sequence $\hat{\boldsymbol{\gamma}}^{(s)}$, $s \in \mathbb{N}$, of MLEs for $\boldsymbol{\gamma}$.

Optimal tests for various test problems concerning a single component γ_1, say, of $\boldsymbol{\gamma}$ are quickly derived by using the findings of Sect. 5.3, since $T_1^{(s)}, \ldots, T_n^{(s)}$ are independent. The conditional distribution of $T_1^{(s)}$ given $T_2^{(s)}, \ldots, T_n^{(s)}$ is thus nothing but the marginal distribution of $T_1^{(s)}$, i.e., a gamma distribution. For instance, a UMPU level-α test for the one-sided test problem

$$H_0 : \gamma_1 \leq \eta \quad \leftrightarrow \quad H_1 : \gamma_1 > \eta$$

for some fixed $\eta \in (0, \infty)$ is given by

$$\varphi(\tilde{\boldsymbol{x}}) = \mathbb{1}_{(0,\chi^2_\alpha(2s))}\left(-2\eta T_1^{(s)}(\tilde{\boldsymbol{x}})\right), \qquad \tilde{\boldsymbol{x}} \in \mathcal{X}^s$$

(see [7]). A UMPU test for the two-sided test problem with null hypothesis $H_0 : \gamma_1 = \eta$ can be obtained by applying Theorem 5.13 leading to a similar situation as in Example 5.9. The corresponding confidence intervals for γ_1 with minimum coverage probabilities of false parameters are shown in [12].

Multivariate test problems with a simple and composite null hypothesis have been studied in the literature. Tests for homogeneity of the parameters including the LR test are shown in [21]. In [9], the Rao score statistic and the Wald statistic have been addressed, the test statistics of which are easily computed, since the Fisher information matrix has diagonal shape (see also [13]). Moreover, confidence regions for $\boldsymbol{\gamma}$ are obtained in [12] by inverting the acceptance regions of tests for a simple null hypothesis. Other confidence regions are constructed in [60] via divergence measures for generalized order statistics. In particular, for $P_1, P_2 \in \mathcal{P}$ with parameter vectors $\boldsymbol{\gamma}^{(1)} = (\gamma_1^{(1)}, \ldots, \gamma_n^{(1)})^t$ and $\boldsymbol{\gamma}^{(2)} = (\gamma_1^{(2)}, \ldots, \gamma_n^{(2)})^t$, say, the Kullback-Leibler divergence $D_{KL}(\boldsymbol{\gamma}^{(1)}, \boldsymbol{\gamma}^{(2)})$ is determined by applying

Lemma 3.37:

$$
\begin{aligned}
D_{KL}(\boldsymbol{\gamma}^{(1)}, \boldsymbol{\gamma}^{(2)}) &= \kappa(\boldsymbol{\gamma}^{(2)}) - \kappa(\boldsymbol{\gamma}^{(1)}) + (\boldsymbol{\gamma}^{(1)} - \boldsymbol{\gamma}^{(2)})^t \pi(\boldsymbol{\gamma}^{(1)}) \\
&= -\sum_{j=1}^{n} \ln(\gamma_j^{(2)}) + \sum_{j=1}^{n} \ln(\gamma_j^{(1)}) - \sum_{j=1}^{n} \frac{\gamma_j^{(1)} - \gamma_j^{(2)}}{\gamma_j^{(1)}} \\
&= \sum_{j=1}^{n} \left[\frac{\gamma_j^{(2)}}{\gamma_j^{(1)}} - \ln\left(\frac{\gamma_j^{(2)}}{\gamma_j^{(1)}}\right) - 1 \right].
\end{aligned}
$$

Obviously, the latter expression depends on component-wise ratios of parameters, only. This finding can be used, e.g., to obtain an exact LR test for the test problem

$$H_0 : \boldsymbol{\gamma} = \boldsymbol{\gamma}^{(0)} \qquad \leftrightarrow \qquad H_1 : \boldsymbol{\gamma} \neq \boldsymbol{\gamma}^{(0)}$$

for fixed $\boldsymbol{\gamma}^{(0)} \in \Xi^*$, which has test statistic $\Lambda_s = 2D_{KL}(\hat{\boldsymbol{\gamma}}^{(s)}, \boldsymbol{\gamma}^{(0)})$ by Theorem 5.16. Based on Cressie-Read divergences, multivariate tests with simple null hypothesis are examined in [60].

An important submodel of generalized order statistics results from the general setting by assuming that successive differences of the parameters are identical, i.e.,

$$\gamma_1 - \gamma_2 = \ldots = \gamma_{n-1} - \gamma_n = m + 1, \text{ say}. \tag{6.24}$$

The model $\mathcal{P}_0 \subset \mathcal{P}$ thus obtained is called m-generalized order statistics, and any distribution in $\mathcal{P}_0$ is determined by specifying m and γ_n. The particular settings $m = \gamma_n - 1$ and $m = -1$ correspond to order statistics and record values, respectively. By utilizing formula (6.24) to rewrite density function $g_{F,\boldsymbol{\gamma}}$ in formula (6.23), $\mathcal{P}_0$ turns out to form a regular EF of order 2 with minimal canonical representation

$$g_{F,m,\gamma_n}(\boldsymbol{x}) = \left(\prod_{j=1}^{n} [(n-j)(m+1) + \gamma_n] \right) e^{mU(\boldsymbol{x}) + \gamma_n V(\boldsymbol{x})} \frac{\prod_{j=1}^{n} f(x_j)}{1 - F(x_n)}$$

and minimal sufficient and complete statistic (U, V) defined by $U(\boldsymbol{x}) = \sum_{j=1}^{n-1} \ln(1 - F(x_j))$ and $V(\boldsymbol{x}) = \ln(1 - F(x_n))$ for $\boldsymbol{x} \in \mathcal{X}$. Here, the natural parameter space is given by

$$\Xi_0^* = \{(m, \gamma_n)^t \in \mathbb{R} \times (0, \infty) : (n-1)(m+1) + \gamma_n > 0\}.$$

More results on this two-parameter EF concerning, in particular, existence, uniqueness, and asymptotic properties of the MLE of $(m, \gamma_n)^t$ can be found in [10].

While the restriction to m-generalized order statistics again results in a regular EF, other assumed relations between the parameters may lead to curved EFs. This is the case, for instance, by connecting $\gamma_1, \ldots, \gamma_n$ via the log-linear link function

$$\ln(\gamma_j) = \tau_1 + \tau_2 z_j\,, \qquad 1 \leq j \leq n\,,$$

where $\tau_1, \tau_2 \in \mathbb{R}$ are link function parameters and $z_1, \ldots, z_n$ are known real numbers, which are not all identical. Properties of curved EFs may then be applied to establish inferential results for $(\tau_1, \tau_2)^t$. For this special link function as well as for other types of link functions, maximum likelihood estimation of the link function parameters is discussed in [59].

References

1. Akahira, M. (2017). *Statistical estimation for truncated exponential families*. Singapore: Springer.
2. Amari, S. I., Barndorff-Nielsen, O. E., Kass, R. E., Lauritzen, S. L., & Rao, C. R. (1987). *Differential geometry in statistical inference*. Hayward: Institute of Mathematical Statistics.
3. Bar-Lev, S. K., & Kokonendji, C. C. (2017). On the mean value parametrization of natural exponential families-A revisited review. *Mathematical Methods of Statistics, 26*(3), 159–175.
4. Barndorff-Nielsen, O. (2014). *Information and exponential families in statistical theory*. Chichester: Wiley.
5. Barndorff-Nielsen, O. E., & Cox, D. R. (1994). *Inference and asymptotics*. Boca Raton: Chapman & Hall.
6. Bauer, H. (2001). *Measure and integration theory*. Berlin: de Gruyter.
7. Bedbur, S. (2010). UMPU tests based on sequential order statistics. *Journal of Statistical Planning and Inference, 140*(9), 2520–2530.
8. Bedbur, S., Beutner, E., & Kamps, U. (2012). Generalized order statistics: An exponential family in model parameters. *Statistics, 46*(2), 159–166.
9. Bedbur, S., Beutner, E., & Kamps, U. (2014). Multivariate testing and model-checking for generalized order statistics with applications. *Statistics, 48*(6), 1297–1310.
10. Bedbur, S., & Kamps, U. (2017). Inference in a two-parameter generalized order statistics model. *Statistics, 51*(5), 1132–1142.
11. Bedbur, S., & Kamps, U. (2019). Testing for equality of parameters from different load-sharing systems. *Stats, 2*(1), 70–88.
12. Bedbur, S., Lennartz, J. M., & Kamps, U. (2013). Confidence regions in models of ordered data. *Journal of Statistical Theory and Practice, 7*(1), 59–72.
13. Bedbur, S., Müller, N., & Kamps, U. (2016). Hypotheses testing for generalized order statistics with simple order restrictions on model parameters under the alternative. *Statistics, 50*(4), 775–790.
14. Berk, R. H. (1972). Consistency and asymptotic normality of MLE's for exponential models. *The Annals of Mathematical Statistics, 43*(1), 193–204.
15. Bhatia, R. (1997). *Matrix analysis*. New York: Springer.
16. Bickel, P. J., & Doksum, K. A. (2015). *Mathematical statistics: Basic ideas and selected topics* (2nd ed., Vol. I). Boca Raton: Taylor & Francis.
17. Billingsley, P. (1995). *Probability and measure* (3rd ed.). New York: Wiley.
18. Billingsley, P. (1999). *Convergence of probability measures* (2nd ed.). New York: Wiley.

S. Bedbur, U. Kamps, *Multivariate Exponential Families: A Concise Guide to Statistical Inference*, SpringerBriefs in Statistics,
https://doi.org/10.1007/978-3-030-81900-2

19. Boyd, S., & Vandenberghe, L. (2004). *Convex optimization*. Cambridge: Cambridge University Press.
20. Brown, L. D. (1986). *Fundamentals of statistical exponential families*. Hayward: Institute of Mathematical Statistics.
21. Cramer, E., & Kamps, U. (2001). Sequential k-out-of-n systems. In N. Balakrishnan & C. R. Rao (Eds.), *Advances in reliability, handbook of statistics* (Vol. 20, pp. 301–372). Amsterdam: Elsevier.
22. Davis, P. J. (1965). Gamma functions and related functions. In M. Abramowitz & I. A. Stegun (Eds.), *Handbook of mathematical functions: With formulas, graphs, and mathematical tables* (pp. 253–294). New York: US Government Printing Office, Dover.
23. Dunn, P. K., & Smyth, G. K. (2018). *Generalized linear models with examples in R*. New York: Springer.
24. Ferguson, T. S. (1967). *Mathematical statistics: A decision theoretic approach*. New York: Academic.
25. Garren, S. T. (2000). Asymptotic distribution of estimated affinity between multiparameter exponential families. *Annals of the Institute of Statistical Mathematics, 52*(3), 426–437.
26. Johnson, N. L., Kemp, A. W., & Kotz, S. (2005). *Univariate discrete distributions* (3rd ed.). New York: Wiley.
27. Johnson, N. L., Kotz, S., & Balakrishnan, N. (1995). *Continuous univariate distributions* (2nd ed., Vol. 2). New York: Wiley.
28. Johnson, N. L., Kotz, S., & Balakrishnan, N. (1997). *Discrete multivariate distributions*. New York: Wiley.
29. Jørgensen, B. (1997). *The theory of dispersion models*. London: Chapman & Hall.
30. Kaas, R., Goovaerts, M., Dhaene, J., & Denuit, M. (2008). *Modern actuarial risk theory* (2nd ed.). Berlin: Springer.
31. Kamps, U. (1995). A concept of generalized order statistics. *Journal of Statistical Planning and Inference, 48*(1), 1–23.
32. Kamps, U. (2016). Generalized order statistics. In N. Balakrishnan, P. Brandimarte, B. Everitt, G. Molenberghs, W. Piegorsch, & F. Ruggeri (Eds.), *Wiley StatsRef: Statistics reference online* (pp. 1–12). Chichester: Wiley.
33. Katzur, A., & Kamps, U. (2016). Classification into Kullback-Leibler balls in exponential families. *Journal of Multivariate Analysis, 150*, 75–90.
34. Katzur, A., & Kamps, U. (2016). Homogeneity testing via weighted affinity in multiparameter exponential families. *Statistical Methodology, 32*, 77–90.
35. Keener, R. W. (2010). *Theoretical statistics: Topics for a core course*. New York: Springer.
36. Kollo, T., & von Rosen, D. (2005). *Advanced multivariate statistics with matrices*. Dordrecht: Springer.
37. Kotz, S., Balakrishnan, N., & Johnson, N. L. (2000). *Continuous multivariate distributions, models and applications* (2nd ed.). New York: Wiley.
38. Krätschmer, V. (2007). The uniqueness of extremum estimation. *Statistics & Probability Letters, 77*(10), 942–951.
39. Lehmann, E. L., & Casella, G. (1998). *Theory of point estimation* (2nd ed.). New York: Springer.
40. Lehmann, E. L., & Romano, J. P. (2005). *Testing statistical hypotheses* (3rd ed.). New York: Springer.
41. Letac, G. (1992). *Lectures on natural exponential families and their variance functions*. Rio de Janeiro: Instituto de Matemática Pura e Aplicada (IMPA).
42. Liese, F., & Miescke, K. J. (2008). *Statistical decision theory: Estimation, testing, and selection*. New York: Springer.
43. Liese, F., & Vajda, I. (1987). *Convex statistical distances*. Leipzig: Teubner.
44. Lindsey, J. K. (2006). *Parametric statistical inference*. Oxford: Clarendon Press.
45. Mardia, K. V., Kent, J. T., & Bibby, J. M. (1979). *Multivariate analysis*. London: Academic.
46. Mies, F., & Bedbur, S. (2020). Exact semiparametric inference and model selection for load-sharing systems. *IEEE - Transactions on Reliability, 69*(3), 863–872.

47. Ng, K. W., Tian, G. L., & Tang, M. L. (2011). *Dirichlet and related distributions: Theory, methods and applications*. Chichester: Wiley.
48. Pardo, L. (2006). *Statistical inference based on divergence measures*. Boca Raton: Chapman & Hall/CRC.
49. Pázman, A. (1986). On the uniqueness of the m.l. estimate in curved exponential families. *Kybernetika, 22*(2), 124–132.
50. Pfanzagl, J. (1994). *Parametric statistical theory*. Berlin: de Gruyter.
51. Rockafellar, R. T. (1970). *Convex analysis*. Princeton: Princeton University Press.
52. Rudin, W. (1976). *Principles of mathematical analysis* (3rd ed.). Auckland: McGraw-Hill.
53. Sen, P. K., & Singer, J. M. (1993). *Large sample methods in statistics: An introduction with applications*. Boca Raton: Chapman & Hall/CRC.
54. Serfling, R. J. (1980). *Approximation theorems of mathematical statistics*. New York: Wiley.
55. Shao, J. (2003). *Mathematical statistics* (2nd ed.). New York: Springer.
56. Sundberg, R. (2019). *Statistical modelling by exponential families*. Cambridge: Cambridge University Press.
57. Vajda, I. (1989). *Theory of statistical inference and information*. Dordrecht: Kluwer.
58. van der Vaart, A. W. (1998). *Asymptotic statistics*. Cambridge: Cambridge University Press.
59. Volovskiy, G., Bedbur, S., & Kamps, U. (2021). Link functions for parameters of sequential order statistics and curved exponential families. *Probability and Mathematical Statistics, 41*(1), 115–127.
60. Vuong, Q. N., Bedbur, S., & Kamps, U. (2013). Distances between models of generalized order statistics. *Journal of Multivariate Analysis, 118*, 24–36.
61. Wei, B. C. (1998). *Exponential family nonlinear models*. Singapore: Springer.
62. Wellek, S. (2010). *Testing statistical hypotheses of equivalence and noninferiority* (2nd ed.). Boca Raton: Chapman & Hall/CRC.
63. Witting, H. (1985). *Mathematische* statistik *I*. Stuttgart: Teubner.

Index

A
Affinely independent, 17

C
Characteristic function, 43
Convex
 function, 29
 hull, 40
 set, 23
Cramér-Rao inequality, 79
Cumulant, 47
Cumulant generating function, 47

D
Distribution
 beta, 12
 binomial, 7
 bivariate normal, 107
 chi-square, 12
 conditional, 47
 Dirichlet, 12
 exponential, 11
 gamma, 11
 geometric, 7
 Good, 8
 inverse gamma, 12
 inverse normal, 11
 joint, 50
 Kemp discrete normal, 8
 Liouville, 12
 log-normal, 12
 marginal, 47
 multinomial, 9
 multivariate normal, 14
 multivariate power series, 9
 negative binomial, 7
 negative multinomial, 117
 normal, 10
 Poisson, 6
 support of, 13
 Wishart, 12
Divergence measure, 60
 Cressie-Read, 61
 Hellinger, 61
 Jeffrey, 61
 Kullback-Leibler, 60
 Rényi, 61

E
Entropy measure, 60
 Shannon, 60
Estimator, 65
 asymptotically efficient, 86
 consistent, 85
 efficient, 81
 maximum likelihood, 69
 strongly consistent, 85
 unbiased, 79
 uniformly minimum variance unbiased, 79
Exponential dispersion model, 53
Exponential family
 canonical representation of, 23
 cumulant function of, 29
 curved, 22
 cut of, 49

S. Bedbur, U. Kamps, *Multivariate Exponential Families: A Concise Guide to Statistical Inference*, SpringerBriefs in Statistics,
https://doi.org/10.1007/978-3-030-81900-2

full, 23
generating measure of, 24
mean value function of, 37
mean value parametrization of, 40
minimal representation of, 17
natural, 24
natural parameter space of, 23
natural parametrization of, 23
order of, 17
regular, 23
steep, 39
truncated, 14
variance function of, 42

F
Fisher information matrix, 58

H
Hypothesis
alternative, 94
of equivalence, 104
null, 94
one-sided, 96
simple, 109
two-sided, 101

L
Likelihood function, 66
Log-likelihood function, 66

M
Maximum likelihood estimate, 66
Moment generating function, 43

N
Neyman-Pearson lemma, 95

P
Parameter
dispersion, 53
identifiable, 21
Product measure, 49

S
Score statistic, 58
Statistic
complete, 55
minimal sufficient, 54
sufficient, 54

T
Test, 93
error probabilities of the first/second kind of, 94
homogeneity, 109
likelihood-ratio, 110
non-randomized, 94
power function of, 94
randomized, 94
Rao score, 111
significance level of, 94
unbiased, 94
uniformly most powerful, 95
uniformly most powerful level-α, 95
uniformly most powerful unbiased level-α, 95
Wald, 111

Printed in the United States
by Baker & Taylor Publisher Services

Printed in the United States
by Baker & Taylor Publisher Services